GOD, BLOOD AND SOCIETY

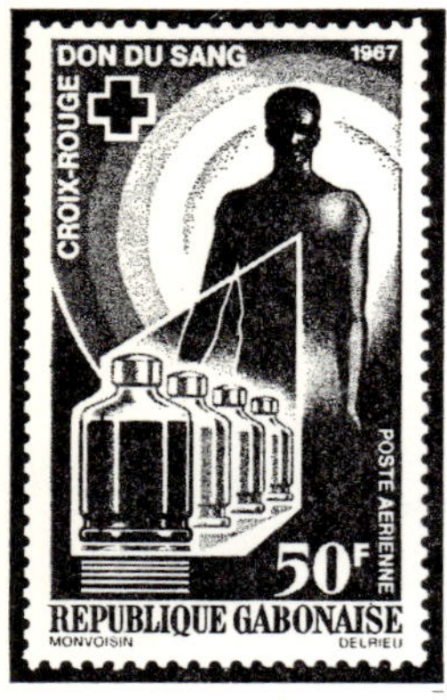

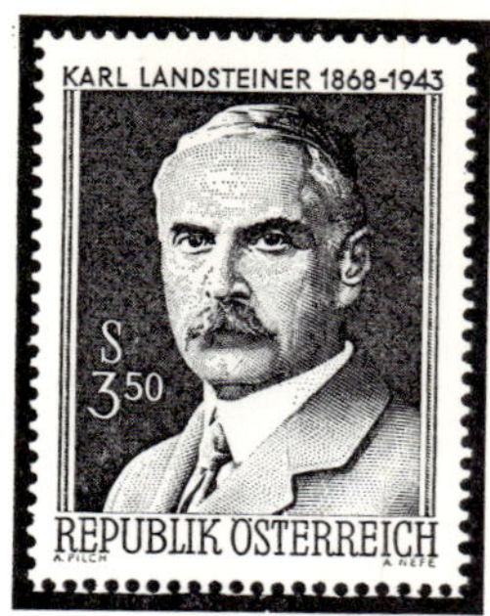

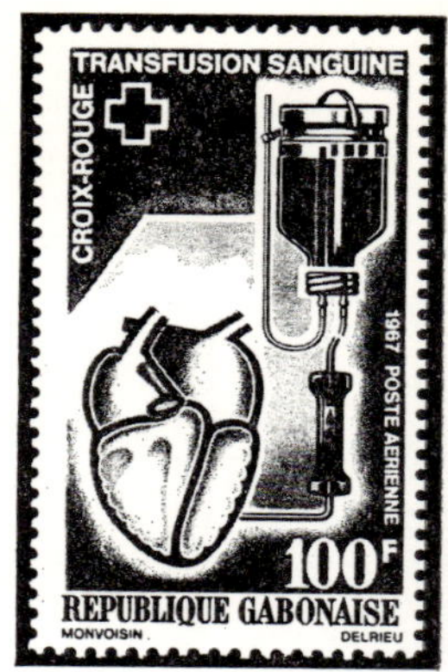

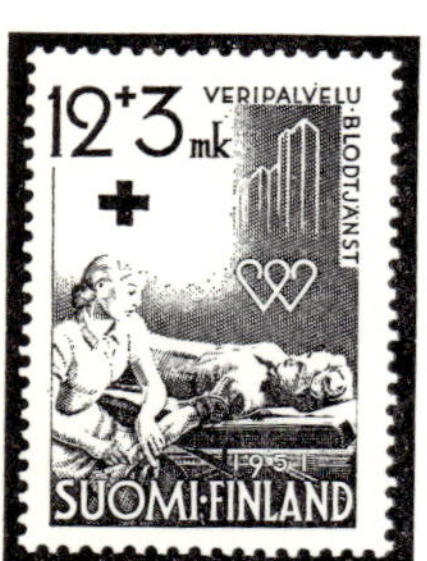

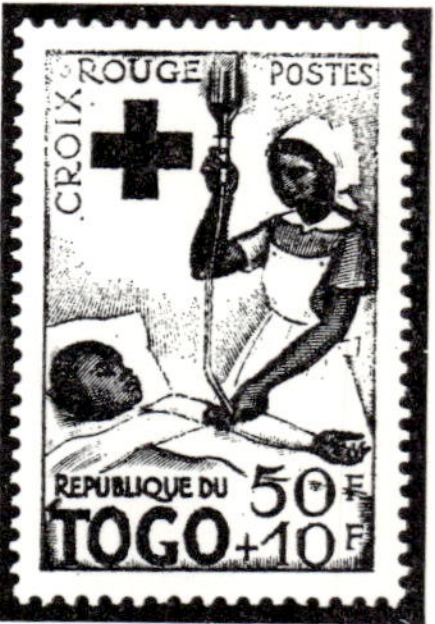

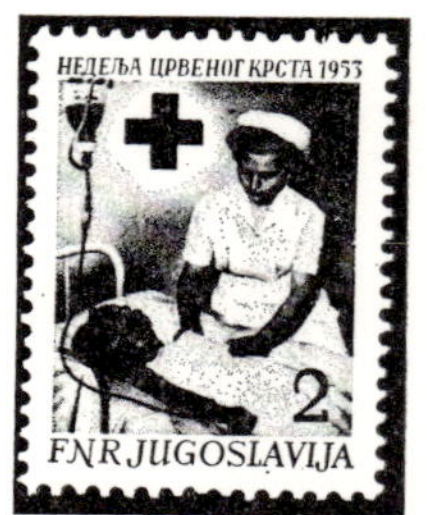

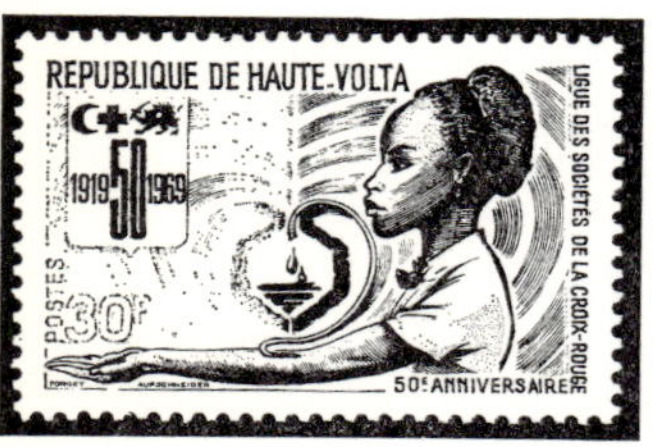

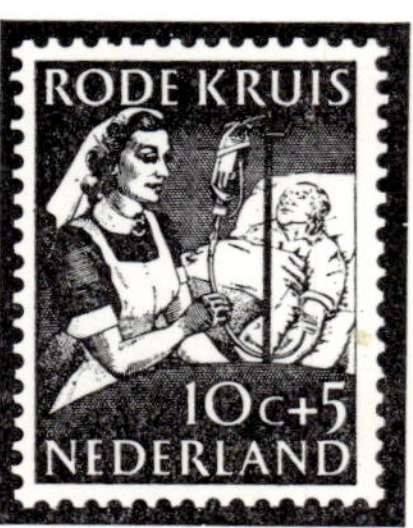

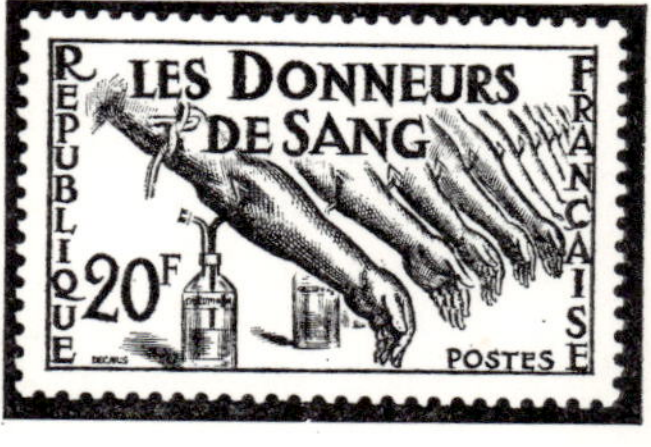

Postage stamps from around the world illustrate the fact that blood transfusion has become a universally accepted practice

GOD, BLOOD AND SOCIETY

A. D. FARR

F.I.M.L.T.

Senior Chief Technician, Aberdeen and N.E. Scotland Blood Transfusion Service Lecturer in Blood Transfusion Techniques, Robert Gordon's Institute of Technology, Aberdeen, and Aberdeen Technical College Diocesan Lay Reader, Episcopal Church in Scotland

IMPULSE BOOKS
ABERDEEN

First published 1972 by

IMPULSE PUBLICATIONS LTD.
28 Guild Street, Aberdeen
Scotland

Printed in Great Britain by Gee & Son, Denbigh

CONTENTS

By the same author

A Laboratory Handbook of Blood Transfusion Techniques

A Synopsis of Blood Grouping Theory and Serological Techniques

The Royal Deeside Line

Stories of Royal Deeside's Railway

The Campbeltown and Machrihanish Light Railway

To Malcolm — and all other 'Rh' babies

ACKNOWLEDGEMENTS

In preparing a study such as this, one is inevitably indebted to a great many people for assistance, advice and information. To all those who have helped in any way it is a pleasure to offer acknowledgement. In particular the following have contributed materially to the book's preparation.

The Very Rev. H. C. Mansbridge and Dr. H. B. M. Lewis, M.R.C.Path., who have read, and offered valuable criticisms of, parts of the manuscript.

The Central Office Manager of the American Association of Blood Banks and Mr. A. R. Midgley of Jehovah's Witnesses have kindly provided much valuable background information.

The Editors of the *Nursing Mirror* and the *Coventry and District Voluntary Blood Donors' Association Newsletter* have consented to the use in Chapter 1 of some material by the author that originally appeared in their publications, and the Secretary of the Medical Defence Union has given permission for the use of some of the material which appears in the M.D.U.'s pamphlet *Consent to Treatment.*

Finally, but by no means least, Mrs. Sheena Wood has translated the author's near-illegible handwriting into typescript, and copied accurately the wide range of technical jargon and detailed Biblical references.

To these, and to all others who have assisted in any way, directly or indirectly, the author offers his most sincere thanks.

PREFACE

In the *Scottish Daily Mail* of June 8, 1965, there appeared a news item: '*Witness refuses blood for dying wife.* Adelaide, Monday. A Jehovah's Witness said to-night he had "no regrets" about refusing a blood transfusion for his 25-year-old wife, who died earlier today giving birth to twins. Mr. Walter Stevens said: "My belief is based on the Scriptures — God forbids the misuse of blood."' From time to time similar items appear in the press and many people wonder what is this belief which allows men and women to die, and teaches them to allow their children to die, rather than receive a blood transfusion?

Writing in the *Bulletin of the American Association of Blood Banks* in March 1960 the Rev. P. L. Swigart coined the word 'Hemophobia' to describe the position, but this is not an accurate term for it is not a phobia, or fear, of blood which motivates those who profess these beliefs. The explanation is very much more complex, and is little understood even by those having to deal with the problem.

In this book an attempt has been made to consider objectively and fairly all the aspects of this problem: medical, theological, legal and ethical. It is all too easy to be swayed by emotion, especially when a child is involved, and to forget that some people hold religious views different from ones own, with just as much honesty and fervour; and with as much right, in a free society, whether we approve of them or not. The purpose of this book is to study these beliefs and their implications.

The conclusions reached in the last chapter may or may not be acceptable to the reader but, having regard to all the arguments and the evidence, the author believes them to be right. If others disagree they at least have in the following pages the evidence upon which that disagreement may be fairly based.

A. DEREK FARR

Rosslynlee,
Cults,
Aberdeen.

I

THE PROBLEM

The use of blood transfusion

Throughout the history of mankind blood has been regarded as a mystic substance to be venerated and regarded with awe. The idea of blood as a therapeutic substance can be traced back to ancient Egypt where the princes bathed in blood as a form of resuscitation and recuperation, while in Rome men would rush into the arena to drink the blood of dying gladiators in the hope of acquiring some of the valour of the victims. Indeed for many centuries the idea of blood as a restorative was wholly restricted to its uses as a draught or for bathing in. In 1492 the frequently quoted 'transfusion' of Pope Innocent VIII was certainly an example of the use of blood as a draught. The aged Pope, following an apoplectic stroke was 'fallen into a kind of somnolency, which was sometimes so profound that the whole court believed him to be dead'. As a means of reviving the stricken pontiff a certain Jewish physician proposed giving to him the blood of a youth. In fact three unfortunate young boys lost their lives in providing blood, but despite this the old man died, and it is recorded that the Jewish physician rapidly disappeared.

It was not until Harvey's publication in 1628 of his then twelve year old discovery of the circulation of the blood that the concept of introducing fluids — including blood — into other bodies arose. Harvey himself had pumped water through the circulation of a dead man, but it was not until 1657 that any important experiments in this line were performed. Dr. (later Sir) Christopher Wren, the famous architect and astronomer, attempted to administer various substances such as ale, wine and opium into the veins of dogs. In a 1667 history of the Royal Society it is said that, 'By this operation creatures were immediately purg'd, vomited, intoxicated, kill'd or revived according to the quality of the liquor injected'. This gave rise to many experiments by the Society, leading to the first transfusion of blood between animals in 1665 by Dr. Richard Lower of Comwall, who was then practising in Oxford.

To a Frenchman, Jean Baptiste Denys, must go the honour of performing the first authenticated transfusion of blood to a human being, in June 1667. Denys bled a boy of about three ounces and gave him in exchange about nine ounces from a lamb. The boy was said to have made a remarkable recovery. In England, Dr. Lower successfully transfused an indigent Bachelor of Divinity, one Arthur Coga, a man described by Pepys as 'cracked a little in his head'. Coga received about twelve ounces of lamb's blood on each of two occasions, and the great diarist records that he appeared unaffected by his ordeal and '. . . finds himself much better since, and as a new man . . .'. Further he records, 'He had but 20s. for his suffering . . .'.

It is interesting to note that in these early years of experimenting the main idea was to attempt to alter the mental outlook of the patient rather than to benefit him physically. Pepys speaks of '. . . many pretty ideas as of the blood of a Quaker to be let into an Archbishop . . .', and there was speculation as to whether a dog transfused with sheep's blood would grow wool and horns, and whether marital discord could be settled by reciprocal transfusions between husband and wife.

Following the initial interest in the procedure, blood transfusion soon fell into the position of little more than an interesting theory. For nearly a century and a half only sporadic experiments took place, until 1818 when an important advance occurred. On December 22 of that year, it fell to Dr. James Blundell, a noted physician, physiologist and obstetrician who was lecturer to Guy's and St. Thomas's Hospitals, to perform the first transfusion of blood from man to man. In all Blundell performed ten transfusions. Of these, two patients were dead before he began and four others were too ill for any treatment to be of avail, but the four other patients all recovered, including apparently hopeless cases of post-partum haemorrhage. In the 80 years following Blundell's work a number of blood transfusions were given in cases of severe blood loss, but the procedure never became really popular.

Transfusions prior to 1900 frequently produced untoward consequences even when using human blood. Rigors, fevers, haemoglobinuria, jaundice, etc. were familiar after-effects which were explained by the brilliant discovery of Karl Landsteiner. This Viennese scientist — who later received a Nobel prize for his discovery — showed that when the blood of different individuals was mixed, agglutination or clumping of the red cells often took place. He divided blood into three groups, which he called A, B and O, on the basis of the agglutinins present in the serum and the antigens on the red cells. In 1902 von DeCastello and Sturli added a fourth group — AB.

Following these discoveries the practice of blood transfusion was now set on a fairly sound scientific basis, and progressed slowly during the following forty years. In 1939 and 1940 Landsteiner — now living in the United States — in conjunction with Dr. A. S. Wiener announced the discovery of the Rh. or Rhesus blood groups. Following some apparently inexplicable fatal cases of severe anaemia in newborn infants they showed that the anaemia was due to an antibody active against the red cells of 85% of white persons. The antigen — called D — responsible is similar to that present in Rhesus monkeys, hence the name given to the group. They showed that where a mother lacked the D antigen and the foetus possessed it (by inheritance from the father) the maternal serum could produce anti-D after a while, which was capable of destroying the foetal red cells and producing severe anaemia and eventual liver damage. The D antigen was the first of the Rh factors to be reported and in the following years a number of others were also reported.

The Rh discovery — of great value in both transfusion and obstetric work — was the first of a steady series of reports of new blood groups. In the first forty years of this century only four group systems had been discovered — ABO, MN and P (by Landsteiner in 1927) and Rh. In the ensuing years further systems have come to light, 14 in all being known at the time of writing. Most of the latter are of but little clinical importance, although of utmost importance to genetecists to whom they are a most valuable guide to the study of inheritance in man.

Since the 1939-45 War, with its great impetus to discoveries in all branches of medical science, the use of blood transfusion has grown enormously until at the present time it has become a commonplace of medical practice. Now that knowledge of the blood groups — incomplete though it is — has made the medical profession aware of some of the great dangers inherent in the practice, standards have improved tremendously until adverse reactions to transfusion are a rarity in those countries with an efficient transfusion service. Blood is used for many purposes, mainly replacing losses due to haemorrhage (both accidental and resulting from surgery) and deficiencies due to disorders of the patient's blood.

One other field in which blood transfusion has advanced has been in the preparation of blood derivatives. The drying of plasma and serum and the production of purified fractions of blood (fibrinogen, thrombin, gamma globulin, etc.) is now a well established science. These fractions are used to treat deficiencies of the specific component in the patient's blood, as well as to provide protection in the form of 'ready-made' antibodies, against certain diseases.

Some religious attitudes to transfusion

In the Bible the word blood occurs four hundred and twenty three times. Considering the veneration given in ancient times to blood as a life-force it is perhaps surprising that the references to it in the sixty-six books, covering some four thousand years of history, are not even more numerous. Those references which do appear in the New Testament mainly allude to the blood of Christ; the Old Testament references are principally to the shedding of blood by violence, and the use of blood for ritual sacrificial purposes. In the latter connection there are a handful of references forbidding the eating of blood — a practice also advised against twice in the Acts of the Apostles. This small collection of prohibitions has in recent years become the cause of much dispute and even loss of life, owing to the interpretation put upon them by the Jehovah's Witnesses — who hold that the practice of blood transfusion is forbidden by God. This belief is carried to the length of allowing one's own death or that of a near relative, rather than agreeing to the receiving of a blood transfusion. Particular notice has been drawn by the press to the death of children whose parents have refused consent to transfusion.

The key texts taken by Jehovah's Witnesses are nearly all to be found in the Pentateuch — the five books of the law which open the Bible. The first pronouncement is contained in Genesis. 'Every moving thing that liveth shall be meat for you; even as the green herb have I given you all things. But flesh with the life thereof, which is the blood thereof, shall ye not eat' (Gen. 9: 3-4). Similarly, 'It shall be a perpetual statute for your generations throughout all your dwellings, that ye eat neither fat nor blood' (Lev. 3: 17). And later in the same book, 'And whatsoever man there be of the house of Israel, or of the strangers that sojourn among you, that eateth any manner of blood: I will even set my face against that soul that eateth blood, and will cut him off from among his people' (Lev. 17: 10). Specifically, the children of Israel were told, 'Only ye shall not eat the blood; ye shall pour it upon the earth as water' (Deut. 12: 16). In the New Testament St. James the Just, in considering whether the gentiles should be required to adhere to Jewish religious law, advised 'that we write unto them, that they abstain from pollutions of idols, and from fornication, and from things strangled, and from blood' (Acts 15: 20), and this was then done (Acts 15: 29).

Now it will be noted that all of these prohibitions (as well as the other repetitions of them which are scattered through the Pentateuch) refer specifically to the *eating* of blood. It was forbidden for the Israelites to eat meat from which the blood had not been drained. The Jehovah's Witnesses relate this eating of blood to blood transfusion, in the sense that they claim both are means of supplying the body with nutriment. They also hold that Deuteronomy 12:16 (quoted above) specifically prohibits the use of blood for any secular purpose whatever, and consequently believe that the practice of transfusion is forbidden by God. This interpretation of the Scriptures raises many problems of ethics, and in particular these are very complex when considering the position of young children who are in need of blood transfusion and who are not in a position to make decisions for themselves.

The legal position

Upon occasion the courts have been involved in problems concerning the transfusion of children, and even of unborn children likely to require exchange transfusion at birth for haemolytic disease of the new-born. In such cases courts have made orders which make the children wards of the court, which then has power to give the necessary consent. In the United States this principle has been taken further with granting of a court order restraining both parents of an unborn child, who were Jehovah's Witnesses, from interfering with medical aid for their child at birth. In Australia the law has been changed following the conviction in 1959 of an English migrant who was a Jehovah's Witness, for manslaughter for failing to give consent for a transfusion to his child who subsequently died. It is not now necessary for a doctor to obtain parents' permission for transfusion in emergency. The position in Britain is less clear. Official advice is that the opinion of a second doctor should be sought before giving a transfusion without consent and that recourse should not be had to the courts, but this still does not prevent the parent from removing a child from medical care, or from subsequently taking civil court proceedings against the doctor concerned. English law has, however, been tested on the principle involved, although not in connection with blood transfusion. The High Court ruled that when refusal of the proper medical care necessary to save a child's life was made deliberately, and in full understanding of the probable consequences, then the person refusing such care is guilty of wilful negligence and, in the case referred to, the defendent was convicted of manslaughter.

The Problem

From what has been so far said it will be obvious that there are two diametrically opposed views of blood transfusion.

The medical profession, and indeed the majority of

laymen of all religions and denominations, regard the practice as a valuable adjunct to treatment of a number of conditions, and as indispensable for saving life in certain cases. The practice is recognised as being hazardous in itself if not properly performed but, with the proper precautions and the functioning of an efficient transfusion service to provide and test the blood, not more hazardous than many other common medical procedures.

The body known as Jehovah's Witnesses view the use of blood for secular purposes as forbidden and its use for transfusion as being directly contrary to the law of God, and therefore entirely unacceptable to themselves.

This clash of opinions about blood transfusion becomes a practical problem when, in the view of orthodox medical practice, a patient who holds views which reject blood himself requires a transfusion in the course of treatment, or even as a lifesaving measure. Popular feeling is often directed to these cases as a result of newspaper publicity, and pressures are brought to bear, sometimes with the force of law, to compel the patient to accept medical advice to which they object. The problem appears far more commonly, and in a more acute form, when the patient is a minor, and legally unable to make his own decision over a matter of conscience. Indeed the greatest concern is usually reserved for cases involving a baby. In these instances there are a number of moral considerations to be taken into account. On the one hand the community has a responsibility to protect those of its number who may not choose for themselves, from the consequences of what majority opinion believes to be wrong or irresponsible behaviour on the part of the parent or guardian; what is frequently overlooked is that every parent or guardian has the right — indeed the duty — to provide for their children that which they believe to be right and necessary for the child's welfare. The decision as to what is right and necessary in any particular case is usually held to be the specific responsibility of the parent. In the case of provision of a blood transfusion parents of the religious persuasion under discussion may consider that such a measure, far from being right is likely to imperil the child's soul ('Whatsoever soul it be that eateth any manner of blood, even that soul shall be cut off from his people.' Lev. 7: 27). It must be remembered that those who subscribe to these beliefs are convinced that they are right, and act as they do in the full knowledge of the possible — even probable — consequences. Has the community in a free country the moral right to over-rule a man's conscience because his beliefs are those of a minority? Or to regard the matter from another viewpoint — has the individual the right to risk the life of himself or his own child in pursuit of beliefs which are not acceptable to the majority of the community?

The problem is not as simple as it might at first appear, and it is only after study of all aspects of it that one may draw conclusions which are logical rather than emotional. Such a study is the purpose of the following chapters.

2

THE MEDICAL POSITION

A brief summary of the history of blood transfusion has already been given. The practice has been developed over the years to a very high standard and while it is undoubtedly potentially hazardous, an efficient blood transfusion service such as exists in most western countries today reduces these hazards to a point where they are no greater than in many other common medical procedures.[16] A high level of safety and reliability exists particularly in those services which are operated free of financial pressures; in which donors provide blood from altruistic motives and patients pay no fee for the provision of blood, nor for its administration. Because it is felt that such a system is conducive to the highest standards of operation, and also because this is the system operated in the United Kingdom, it is the one to be described. Notes will, however, be included indicating some possible dangers peculiar to a service that is not entirely free from financial considerations for either donor or patient.

The composition of blood

Blood consists of a fluid called plasma, which contains in suspension red cells (erythrocytes), white cells (leucocytes) and platelets (thrombocytes). The function of the red cells is basically to transport gasses. The cells are bi-concave discs measuring 7.2 microns × 2.1 microns (1 micron = 1/1,000mm.), and consist of a membrane containing a solution of a substance called haemoglobin (Hb) which is chemically a compound of iron and protein and which, combined with oxygen gives blood its red colour. The haemoglobin is capable of taking up gases and, in the course of circulating round the body, carries oxygen from the lungs to the tissues, and carbon dioxide back to the lungs. The leucocytes are primarily part of the body's defence system against infection and are capable of ingesting bacteria. Platelets are part of the very complicated chain reaction which causes blood to clot when shed. Normal blood will contain roughly 4.5 to 5.5 million red cells in every cubic millimetre, as well as 7,000 - 12,000 white cells and about 150,000 - 400,000 platelets. The plasma is a complex fluid which is about 91% water, and contains in solution a number of inorganic salts and organic substances — mainly proteins. Of these latter, albumin, gamma globulin and fibrinogen are the most important together with a number of clotting factors of which Factor VIII (antihaemophilic-factor — AHF) may be particularly mentioned.

Source of blood

Blood is taken from healthy donors of either sex between 18 and 65 years of age, who are not currently suffering from any infection and who do not suffer from any of a number of conditions which may be either (*a*) transmissable by blood, (*b*) contagious, or (*c*) potentially harmful to themselves if they act as blood donors.

The age limits are those prescribed in Great Britain and are intended to act as a general safeguard against removal of blood from adolescents during a period of growth and development, or from older people who generally are in less perfect health, and who may regenerate blood more slowly, and be more susceptible to infection.

The exclusion of donors suffering from current infections or contagious conditions is an obvious safety measure designed to protect donor, patient, and bleeding staff and other donors with whom the individual may come into contact. Certain conditions may prove harmful to the donor if he gives blood — obvious examples are heart disease, epilepsy (risk of injury if a fit occurs while a needle is in the donor's vein), history of strokes, etc. There are only four types of condition which are normally transmissable directly by transfusion: syphilis, malaria, allergies (temporarily) and jaundice.

In the case of syphilis (and this includes yaws and other spirochaetal infections) a number of tests exist which can detect antibodies formed by the individual in response to the infection. It is true that these antibodies are not detectable in the primary stages of infection, but the spirochaete responsible will not survive more than about four days at the storage temperature of blood (4-6°C)[1] and as comparatively little blood is used within this age period the risk of accidental transfusion of spirochaetal infected blood is minimal. In fact the contraction of syphilis following transfusion is now virtually non-existent. The tests usually performed on all donor bloods for spirochaetal antibodies may be used either singly or in combination with each other.

Donors giving a history of recurring allergies are generally not accepted, nor are those who have suffered an attack of malaria (or other plasmodial infection) during the previous five years, or who have returned during that time from an area where malaria is endemic. Donors with a malarial history more than five years previously may be accepted for use of their blood in the preparation of plasma or plasma fractions only, as any 'dormant' plasmodia will in any case be found only in the red cells.

Homologous serum jaundice is a very dangerous virus infection which is readily transmissable by means of very small volumes of blood, and which may be fatal. Due to the difficulty of distinguishing between a history of jaundice due to this virus and one of a purely obstructive nature — which is not transmissable — it has for many years been usual to reject all donors with any history of jaundice at all. More recently a series of tests has become available to supplement these histories. A virus particle known as the Australia, or Hepatitis Associated, Antigen has been demonstrated. The precise nature and significance of this particle is still not fully understood, but it is clear that where it exists in the blood of an individual then that blood is potentially capable of transmitting serum jaundice. Tests for the presence of the Australia Antigen are far from perfect, and the significance of a negative reaction or of a reaction demonstrating the presence of an antibody active against the antigen must be appreciated; such blood is not necessarily free of hepatitis risk. What these tests do, however, is clearly to indicate a number of blood donors whose blood carries the risk of transmitting hepatitis, and exclusion of these from the donor panel considerably improves the safety of blood transfusion. In Scotland, virtually all blood donors are now tested for

Australia Antigen and antibody, and the testing is becoming widespread elsewhere, despite considerable difficulties in obtaining suitable reagents and in the technical performance of the tests. In New York State it has been made a compulsory requirement that all blood supplied for transfusion shall have been so tested.

It is here that some of the advantages of using non-paid donors may be seen It is extremely difficult to detect with any reliability carriers of hepatitis and of malaria. Considerable reliance may have to be placed upon the donor's honesty in signing a declaration of freedom from these conditions. With the purely altruistic donor this is possible. With a paid donor, who would by such an admission forfeit his payment, it is entirely unrealistic. It is indeed an unfortunate fact that in countries where paid donors are used these are often recruited from the dregs of society,[2] and amongst people who find this their only source of livelihood.[3]

In order that donors are not used who are themselves anaemic a haemoglobin estimation is performed and only those donors accepted who have a minimum level of 85% (females) or 90% (males).[4] These figures are well within normal limits.

Collection

Blood is collected by insertion of a needle into one of the veins of the antecubital fossa — the 'inside' of the elbow — and allowing the blood to flow *via* a length of rubber or plastic tubing into a glass bottle (or a specially prepared plastic bag) which contains an anticoagulant / preservative mixture; this solution both prevents clotting and also helps to preserve the blood during storage. The blood may flow either by gravity, in which case there must be an adequate outlet for air displaced from the bottle, or the container may possess a vacuum equal to or greater than the amount of blood to be collected, in which case an air outlet may not be necessary. In the case of plastic bags, as the bag is empty of air, there is no need for either air outlet or vacuum. The standard volume of blood collected at each donation in this country is 420 ml. (about three quarters of a pint) and donors are never bled more frequently than once every three months, more usually once every six months. In countries where donors are paid for their services it is not uncommon for them to present themselves at very much more frequent intervals, possibly at different centres. This practice may readily lead to a state of chronic anaemia in the donor if adequate haemoglobin estimations are not carried out. This is of course a further disadvantage, and even danger, of a 'commercial' transfusion service. One donation represents about eight per cent of the blood volume — a loss which is very readily tolerated by a normal healthy adult.[1]

The apparatus used for collection of blood, including the container and anticoagulant, is sterilized before use and constant checks on the efficiency of the sterilizing process are carried out. There is only one serious complication which may arise in blood donation — air embolism. If blood is collected into a bottle by gravity and for any reason the air outlet from the bottle becomes blocked it is possible that a positive air pressure may build up in the bottle and, at the end of the donation, air may pass through the taking set into the donor's vein. The possibility of such an accident is well appreciated and a technique is used in bleeding which completely eliminates the risk. As a matter of interest as much as 300ml. (about half a pint) of air has been recorded as entering a vein, the patient recovering completely within ten minutes.[5] In order that donors do not walk out from making their donation and suffer an accident due to any transient faintness, a resting period of twenty minutes following donation is insisted upon, during which time they are served with refreshments.

It only remains to add that since the inception of the National Health Service many decorations for having given 50 or more donations of blood have been awarded in Great Britain, as well as a great many more for giving 25 or more donations. More than 1,000,000 donations are given to the British transfusion services annually. No case of ill health or disease attributable to repeated blood donation has yet been reported.

Storage[1]

The solution into which blood is collected is known as A.C.D. or acid-citrate-dextrose.

The dextrose is purely to help preservation, by replacing dextrose utilised on storage in the donor blood, and the acid sodium citrate prevents clotting.

Citrate may itself be toxic if administered in very large doses, but as it is excreted very rapidly by the body sufficiently large concentrations to prove toxic never build up in normal practice. When exceptionally large volumes of citrated blood are used during a short period, as in exchange transfusion in the newborn, the effects of citrate toxicity are readily prevented by routine administration of calcium gluconate[1]; alternatively another anticoagulant such as heparin may be used.

Prior to use blood is stored at 4-6°C (38-42°F) for a period of not more than 21 days.[4] At these temperatures the survival of the red cells is optimal, as well as the risk of bacterial multiplication being minimal. An occasional bacterium will, despite every precaution, occasionally find its way into a bottle of blood and if it is not immediately destroyed by the bactericidal properties of fresh blood — as is most probable —the low storage temperature will prevent it from multiplying. Occasional single bacteria are not dangerous in transfusion — only moderately heavy growths cause harm.[1] The necessity for limiting the storage period to 21 days is due to the fact that blood is a living tissue, and the cells are constantly dying. The average life of a red cell is about 100 to 120 days, so that after about 21 days of storage a number of the cells in a bottle will be effete. If blood which appears satisfactory is transfused after more than 21 days no harm will generally result, but neither will any benefit ensue; most of the cells will be rapidly eliminated from the patient's circulation.

One further potential hazard remains with stored blood. Shortly after storage commences there is a gradual 'shift' of potassium from within the red cells into the plasma. After 10-15 days the levels of potassium in the plasma are markedly raised and, as with citrate, very large volumes of such blood given over a short period may possibly prove dangerous in some individuals. The simple solution is that only blood less than 10 days old (preferably less than seven) is used in such cases.

The blood groups[6,7]

One of the greatest hazards in blood transfusion is connected with the blood groups. It must at once be said that this is a very complicated subject and no more than a very brief resumé of the problems can be attempted here. For anyone wishing to obtain more detailed information the books referred to (6, 7) may be consulted.

It was discovered around 1900 that all individuals belong to four groups, depending on the presence of one or other, both or neither of two factors (antigens) on the red cell surface; these were called A and B. Complementary to these factors there are substances called antibodies present in the plasma. Every individual possesses the antibodies corresponding to whichever antigens he does not have on the red cells. Thus, if a person has the A antigen on the cells he will have anti-B in his plasma. The position is summarized below.

Red cells	Plasma
O	Anti-A and Anti-B
A	Anti-B
B	Anti-A
AB	No antibodies

Now if plasma containing anti-A is mixed in a test tube with blood carrying A antigens, the red cells carrying the antigens will be clumped together into large clusters; this process is called agglutination. Occasionally with some potent antibodies the red cells may break down completely — the process of haemolysis. If such a mixture should take place in the circulation — as may for example happen if a group B patient were given a transfusion of group A blood — the transfused cells affected by the patient's antibody are removed from the circulation by either the liver or the spleen, and the resulting products will probably cause sufficient damage to the excretory organs (the kidneys) to cause a very severe illness, possibly death. It will thus be seen that it is of prime importance that a patient is given only blood of his own group. The ABO groups, however, are not the whole story.

In 1939-40 a blood group system called Rh (Rhesus) was discovered. It was named after the rhesus monkey in whose blood the Rh antigen was first discovered. Very simply, everyone either has or has not the Rh antigen, and so the terms applied were Rh-positive and Rh-negative. There is virtually no such thing as a naturally occuring Rh antibody, as is the case with the ABO groups. If, however, a person who lacks the Rh antigen (Rh-negative) is transfused with blood which carries it (Rh-positive) that individual may gradually form anti-Rh in their plasma as a response, in much the same way that an injection of (killed) typhoid organisms causes the formation of protective anti-typhoid antibodies in a process of immunisation. Not only may anti-Rh be formed by transfusion however. If an Rh-negative woman is pregnant with an Rh-positive baby — and as blood group factors are inherited this may not infrequently happen — it is possible for some of the baby's Rh-positive blood to leak into the mother's circulation and immunise her, causing the formation of anti-Rh in the same way as if she had received a transfusion of Rh-positive blood. In either case the process of immunisation has no immediate effect but if on a subsequent occasion, the anti-Rh having been once formed, the patient receives a further transfusion of Rh-positive blood then there may be an adverse reaction similar to that already described with the ABO groups. Having once been formed, antibodies of this type remain in the patient's circulation more or less indefinitely. Unfortunately, in the case of women of child-bearing age there may be further complications. If a woman, having from any cause formed anti-Rh, again becomes pregnant with an Rh-positive child, then the mother's Rh-antibody may pass into the infant's circulation and destroy its Rh-positive red cells in the same way that it would destroy transfused Rh-positive red cells. This leads to the baby being born more or less severely anaemic, and sometimes so dangerously affected that it may only survive a short time, or even be stillborn. This condition, known as haemolytic disease of the newborn, was at one time very frequently fatal but is nowadays nearly always satisfactorily treated by blood transfusion.

Rhesus immunisation as a result of pregnancy can now be prevented with a high degree of success. Women forming anti-Rh do so nearly always as a result of a trans-placental haemorrhage at delivery. Women at risk following the delivery of a Rh-positive baby are given an injection of anti-D immunoglobulin. This material — a blood product — is in effect a very concentrated dose of pre-formed anti-Rh antibody. Its effect is to destroy any of the baby's cells which have entered the maternal circulation, before they can immunise the mother. Being a 'foreign' protein in the mother's circulation the immunoglobulin itself will be fairly quickly eliminated so that by the time of her next pregnancy the mother's blood is free of injected anti-Rh, and has not formed any as a result of immunisation by her baby's red cells. Widespread use of this form of protection will probably result in haemolytic disease of the newborn being almost completely eliminated within the next twenty years or so, but it will be noted that this end can only be achieved by the administration of another blood product.

At the beginning of this section the reader was warned that blood groups are a complicated subject, and it is at this point that this becomes obvious.

Rh is not a simple, single factor. Since the original discovery in 1939, a number of other related factors have been discovered, and these may be found in a bewildering number of permutations. At the present time nearly three hundred different Rh types may theoretically be recognised. Furthermore the ABO and Rh blood group systems are merely the two most important of fourteen known at present. Some of the other twelve systems are as 'simple' as the ABO groups, others are more complicated; a few are not of clinical significance in causing reactions to transfusions or haemolytic disease of the newborn, but most of them may be.

The position is yet further complicated by the fact that blood group antibodies do not all act in the same way. A number of different laboratory techniques need to be employed to demonstrate them and it is probable that a few antibodies exist which cannot be detected by any method known at present.

In view of the near impossibility of transfusing any blood which is exactly identical to that of the recipient, a cross-match test is performed prior to every transfusion. This consists of testing the patient's plasma against the red cells of every potential donor, having

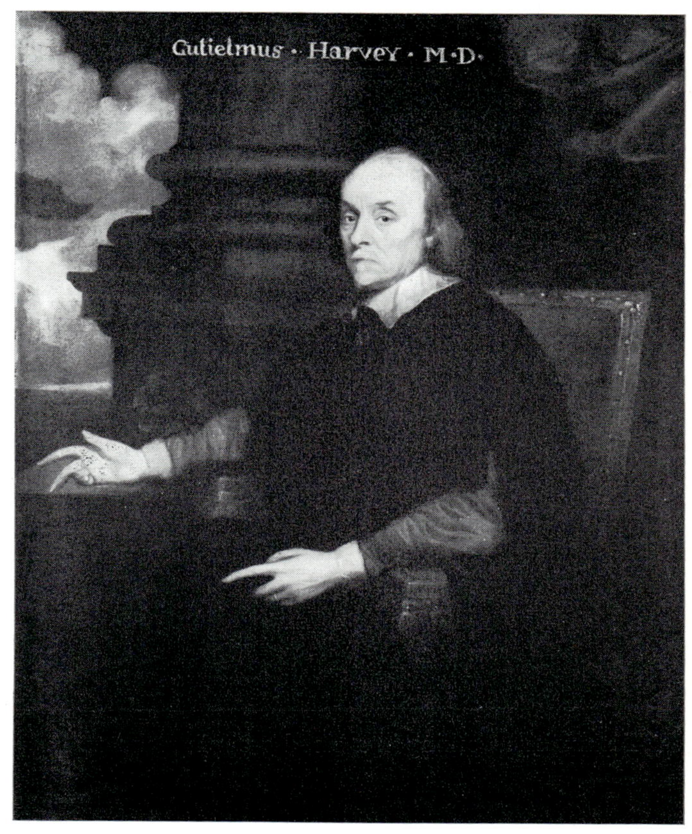

William Harvey (1578-1657)
The discoverer of the circulation of the blood.
(By permission of the Royal College of Physicians, London)

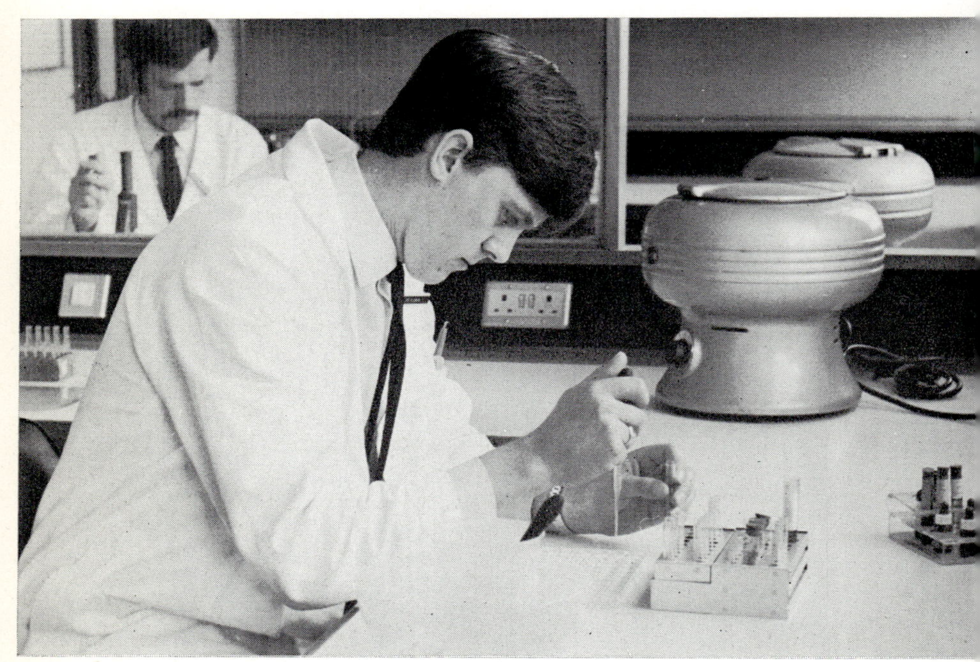

Technicians working in a blood grouping laboratory

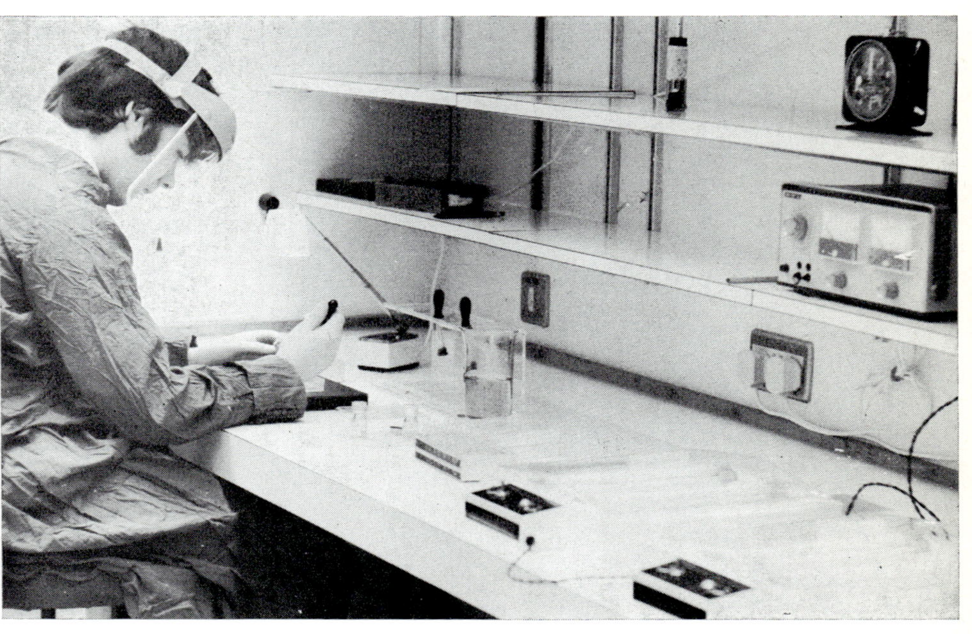

Testing donor blood for the Australia (Hepatitis Associated) Antigen

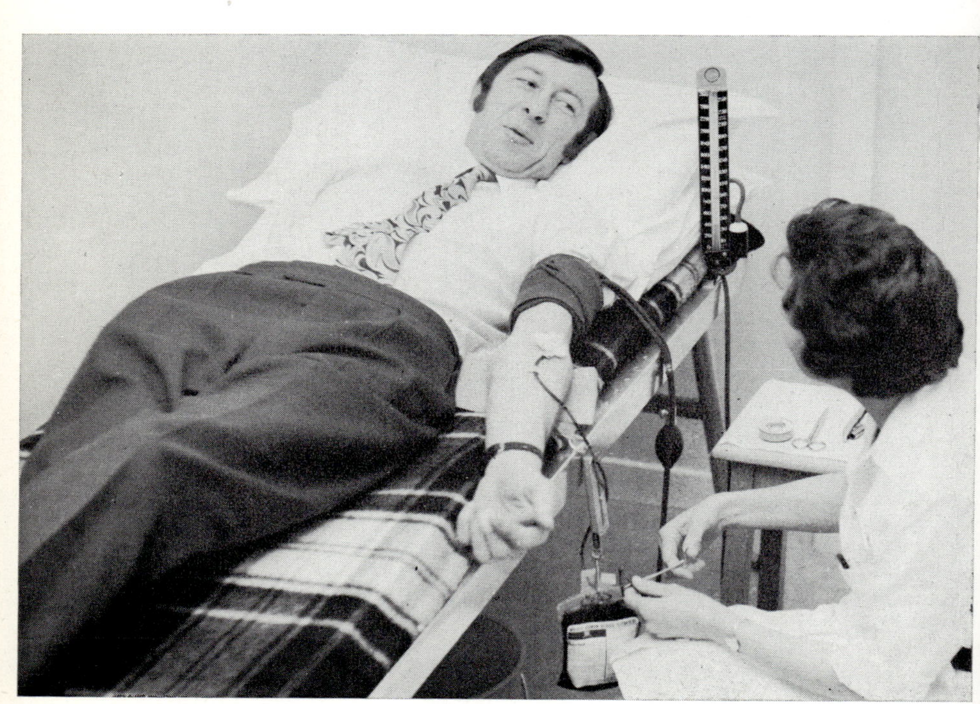

Giving a blood donation

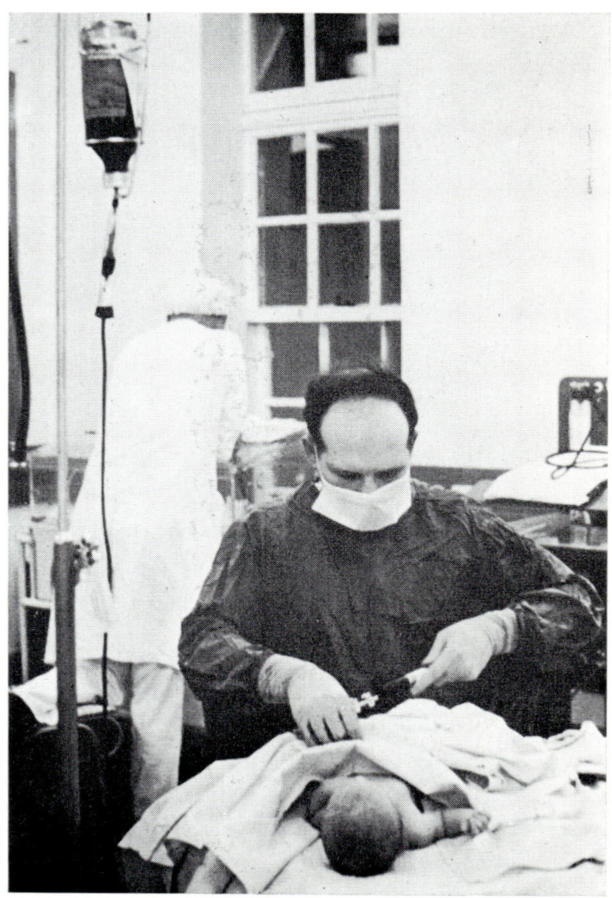

A newborn baby receiving an exchange transfusion for Rhesus haemolytic disease

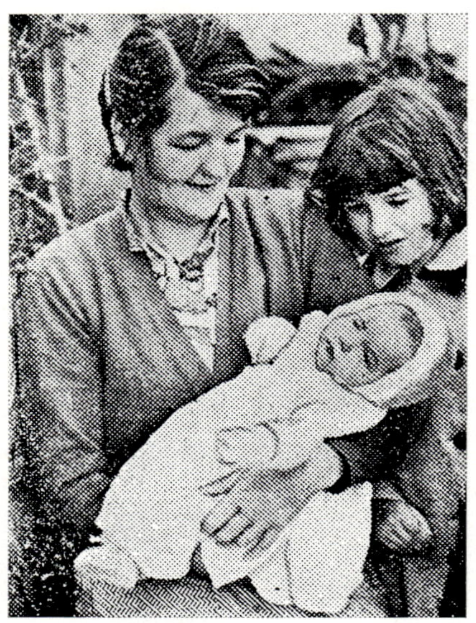

Mrs. V. T. of Gloucestershire who survived a severe haemorrhage following the birth of her fifth child. She was given thirty-five pints of blood in six hours. She is now a blood donor herself.

(Photograph by permission of The Bristol Evening Post)

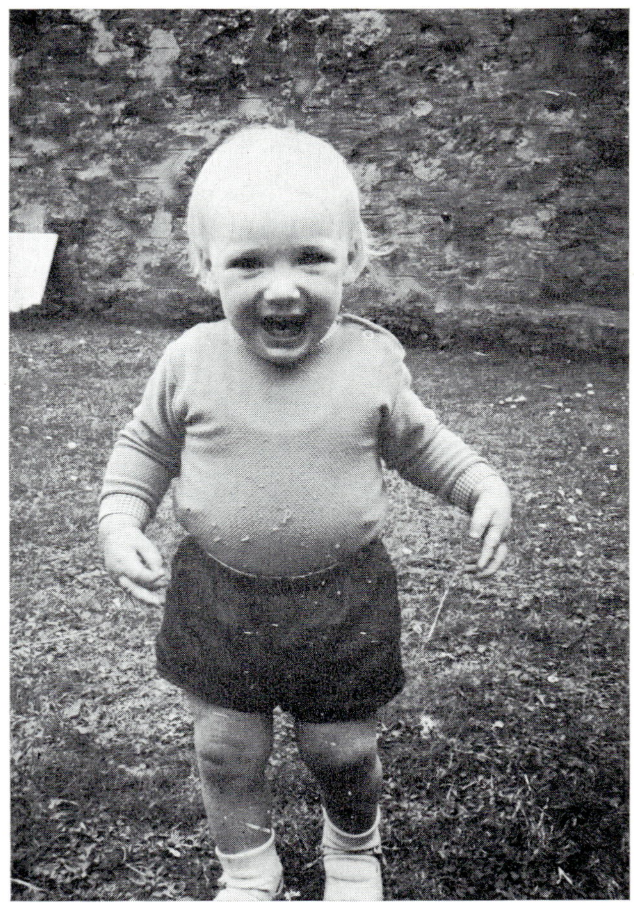

Malcolm was a 'Rhesus baby' who needed three complete exchange transfusions during his first week of life. His mother had lost two of her previous children as a result of this disorder.

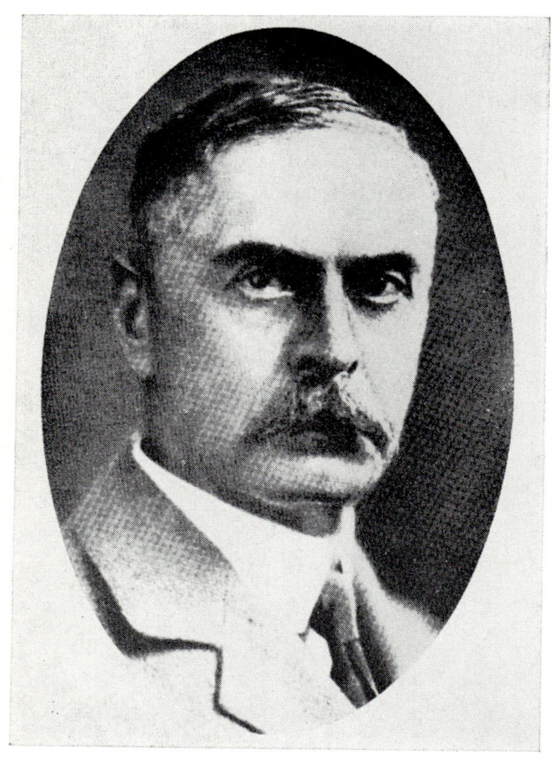

Karl Landsteiner (1868-1943)
The discoverer of the blood groups.
(From Pollack, O. J.: Grouping, Typing and Banking of Blood, 1951. Courtesy of Charles C. Thomas, Publisher, Springfield, Illinois)

Except where otherwise stated, photographs are by the author first ensured that the ABO and Rh groups are the same. The test is performed using several different techniques so that if any incompatibility exists it will be demonstrated. Adequate tests take several hours to perform. It must be stressed that the risk of immunising a patient by means of transfusion is, outside the Rh system, very small. The cross-match itself will of course only detect existing antibodies.

It will be obvious that the selection of blood for transfusion to individual patients is a skilful and highly responsible task, and any reputable transfusion service safeguards the patient by ensuring that it is only undertaken by experienced and skilled serologists. This particular task calls for special training and may be performed by suitably experienced doctors or technicians. Possession of a medical degree or a registerable qualification in medical laboratory technology is not in itself sufficient.

Use of blood products

The components of blood which are generally used separately for therapeutic or prophylactic purposes are as follows.

Concentrated red cells. In cases of anaemia, where it is desired to raise the number of red cells in the circulation without increasing total blood volume excessively, it is usual to transfuse red cells from which most of the plasma — citrate mixture has been removed, thus reducing the volume of each donation by about 50%.

Washed packed cells. In cases such as paroxysmal nocturnal haemoglobinuria the patient's red cells are destroyed by a substance found in normal plasma. In these cases concentrated cells prepared as above are further ' washed ' with a sterile solution of salt (normal saline) to remove all the plasma before transfusion.

Platelet preparations. Various concentrations of platelets in their own plasma can be prepared for transfusion to patients who have a platelet deficiency.

Plasma. The fluid portion of blood may be separated, pooled to neutralise blood group antibodies, and dried. In the dry state plasma may be stored for many years, and reconstituted with distilled water when needed. It is used in cases of severe burns and oligaemic shock when the patient has lost plasma from the circulation into the tissues, so that the blood has become too concentrated, and the total blood volume too low. It is also used as a general emergency fluid to replace blood loss when whole blood is not available.

Plasma fractions. By a chemical process of precipitation plasma proteins may be fractionated and collected as pure preparations. They are either dried like plasma or issued as solution in a suitable buffered fluid.[8]

Albumin is used for much the same purposes as whole plasma. It is, however, free of the risk of transmitting jaundice.

Gamma globulin (Normal Immunoglobulin) may be used either as a supply of this protein in patients in whom it is deficient, or for the prophylaxis of various virus diseases such as measles and rubella and in infective hepatitis. As all the antibodies the individual forms against infection consist of gamma globulins, a purified form of this protein will contain high concentrations of ready-made antibodies.

Fibrinogen is a substance which is essential in forming a blood clot. Patients deficient in this who have a haemorrhage may bleed to death from lack of fibrinogen and a concentrated preparation is administered in such cases.

Anti-haemophilic-factor is another substance which is essential for blood clotting. In the hereditary condition of haemophilia this is deficient and the patient can bleed to death from even a small cut or bruise. Dental extraction is a major operation in such people, who are nearly always males. In order to provide cover for such necessary surgery, as well as to stop bleeding in accidental haemorrhage, purified AHF may be used.

More commonly a crude preparation of Factor VIII (the anti-haemophilic factor) is used; this is known as cryo-precipitate and is prepared by snap-freezing fresh plasma and then thawing it slowly at 4°C and collecting the resultant precipitate.

Blood 'substitutes'

A number of chemical preparations have been evolved over the years to act as artificial substitutes for blood (or rather for plasma, as it is not possible to imitate the gas-transport function of red cells). As these substances contain no proteins the term 'substitute' is incorrect and the proper expression is plasma volume expanders. Only one such substance has proved of value — Dextran — all the others are either too transient in action to be of any value, or are stored permanently in the tissues and may be carcinogenic. In particular PVP (polyvinyl-pyrollidone) which is sometimes suggested by the Jehovah's Witnesses as an alternative to blood is not now used owing to the risks of such retention. Normal saline (0.9% sodium chloride in distilled water) which they also sometimes recommend is of little use as the effect on blood volume is extremely transient. In addition, large volumes of saline lead to an increase in extravascular fluid which may cause the syndrome of post-operative drowning.[9]

Dextran is a preparation of a depolymerised polysaccharide which is very effective in maintaining blood volume for a reasonable length of time and appears to have a similar action to plasma.[1] The volume given per patient should be limited to 1 litre owing to the possibility of dangerous over-dilution of the plasma proteins with larger volumes. That Dextran is not entirely incapable of causing adverse reactions is shown by reports of abnormally prolonged bleeding time and allergic reactions following its use.[10]

Reasons for transfusion

Basically there are two main reasons why transfusions of blood or plasma are given — haemorrhage and anaemia. In addition various blood fractions may be used in conditions where these are deficient in the patient (e.g. the use of A.H.F. in haemophilia).

Haemorrhage

The average individual can, in health, withstand the loss of a litre or more of blood with few if any ill effects.[1] In a wounded patient, however, the effects of blood loss may be more serious. The main effects of haemorrhage are reductions in venous pressure and in blood volume. A normal person will replace a lost volume of as much as 1 litre of blood within about 36 hours,[11] but the haemoglobin concentration (reflecting the number of red cells) takes three to four weeks to regain normal levels after the loss of only 400ml. of blood.[12]

In general, blood transfusion is necessary following haemorrhage only when large volumes of blood have been lost and the systolic blood pressure is dangerously reduced. In such cases transfusion will be necessary to save life. Once a transfusion has been started there is no merit in stopping it if, after a small volume has been given, the patient appears improved, as the blood volume will still be low and the patient still in danger.[1] On the other hand care is necessary that the circulation is not overloaded. Blood loss is difficult to measure due to loss into the tissues as well as from the wound, and it is for this reason that blood pressure is generally used as an index of the patient's need for transfusion. Transfusions of only one unit of blood (540ml.) to an adult are hardly ever justified in the face of the inherent hazards of blood transfusion, as the loss of such a volume is scarcely ever critical, and large blood losses require larger replacements.

Anaemia

Anaemia may be due either to a reduction in the number of circulating red cells or to a reduction in the amount of haemoglobin carried in a normal number of cells. Generally speaking blood transfusion should only be used to correct anaemia if this cannot be done by administration of haematinic drugs (iron preparations, vitamin B_{12} etc.), or if a rapid increase in red cell volume is essential (e.g. anaemia produced by haemorrhages which will probably recur, severe anaemia in a patient required to undergo emergency surgery, etc.).[1] The only types of chronic anaemia unlikely to respond to other treatment are generally those in which there is a deficiency in red cell production (e.g. aplastic anaemia) or abnormal red cell destruction (e.g. paroxysmal nocturnal haemoglobinuria). The latter type of anaemia frequently shows only transient improvement with transfusion. In patients with very profound anaemias transfusion may prove fatal by causing circulatory overloading, and is thus better avoided if other treatment is possible.[1]

In haemolytic disease of the newborn blood transfusion has three objectives. It is of course aimed at raising the haemoglobin level (i.e. treating the anaemia) but it has two more important functions. Excessive destruction of the infant's red cells leads to gross jaundice due to the presence in the plasma of a pigment called bilirubin. This jaundice is liable, if left untreated, to lead to a permanent damage of the central nervous system, called kernicterus. This condition is usually fatal but if the infant survives it will suffer permanent mental damage and retardation.[1] In order to remove the excess bilirubin and at the same time remove the maternal antibodies which are causing the red cell destruction, and also correct the anaemia, exchange (or replacement) transfusion is carried out. In this procedure the entire circulating blood volume of the infant is replaced with fresh blood of a type which is compatible with the baby and with the maternal antibody which is causing the condition. Such exchange transfusions may need to be repeated several times but eventually the vast majority of affected children survive without permanent damage, and subsequently develop normally.

A proportion of affected children will not survive the full term of pregnancy and will die of anaemia if untreated. There is a limit to the degree of prematurity at which a child can be delivered with hope of survival and in severe cases a technique is now available to give such babies a simple (i.e. not an exchange) transfusion while still in the mother's uterus. This technique aims at maintaining the haemoglobin level until it is possible to deliver the baby prematurely and perform an exchange transfusion.

Administration

A brief note on the method of administering blood is of importance, as will be realised when reading Chapter 4.

An apparatus is used which enables the blood to be given without the necessity for opening the bottle. A two-level needle assembly is inserted through the rubber closure of the blood bottle, and the bottle is inverted. The upper end of the assembly in this inverted position acts as an airway, leading via a length of tubing to an air filter; the lower end is attached to a long length of rubber or plastic tubing, in the length of which is included at some point a filter, a 'drip counter' device with which the rate of flow may be measured, and a regulating device with which the flow-rate may be controlled. The tubing terminates in a needle which is inserted into a convenient vein, usually in the patient's arm. (Occasionally blood has been transfused directly into an artery if the rate of blood loss in a severe haemorrhage was very great.) When blood is being given from plastic bags the apparatus is similar but has a single outlet instead of the two-level needle assembly, as there is no need for an air outlet. The blood flows by gravity from the raised inverted bottle and mixes with the patient's blood already passing through the vein. In case of very rapid blood loss the transfusion may be speeded up by applying a positive pressure to the air-way of the bottle, although this procedure is hazardous in that an air embolism may develop if a close continuous watch is not kept on the level of blood in the bottle.

The essential point to be noted for the purposes of this study is that the transfused blood enters directly into the patient's own circulation.

In the case of transfusions of unborn babies in the uterus a different approach is taken. It is known that if red cells are introduced into the peritoneal cavity of the abdomen they will be absorbed intact, via the lymphatic system, into the circulation. Use is made of this by introducing a fine tube into the mother's uterus and into the baby's peritoneal cavity, guided by X-ray pictures. Red cells are then dripped through this tube in similar fashion to an ordinary transfusion. Once again it should be noted that intact red cells enter the patient's circulation unaltered.

Use and abuse of transfusion

It may appear to the reader that an excessive amount of space and detail have been expended on this chapter.

The reason for this is that the Jehovah's Witnesses, while maintaining their stand against blood transfusion primarily on religious grounds, nevertheless devote 40% of their booklet on the subject[2] to medical objections to the practice. There is no doubt that blood transfusion can be a hazardous procedure if not properly performed, nor that it does tend to be used with unwonted freedom in some cases. It is in order that the number of complications which undeniably can arise may be appreciated that so much detail has been given. In their opposition to transfusion on medical grounds the Witnesses undeniably have a case, insofar as, like any other medical procedure it can be dangerous and it can be abused.[13]

In cases of haemorrhage, transfusion is generally necessary as a life-saving measure in only a comparatively few instances where very massive blood loss has occurred. Even in planned surgery blood loss is not often sufficient to make transfusion necessary, even though it may often be desirable. In many cases the use of dextran will suffice. Even in open heart surgery with a heart-lung machine it is possible with the latest apparatus, to perform surgery without blood. The machine being primed with a solution of dextrose, although it is necessary to run the patient's own blood through the machine. While such surgery is possible it undeniably involves a much greater risk than where blood is used. In the treatment of anaemia there is little doubt that the use of blood is often resorted to when it is not necessary to save life, although in some cases it may be the only life-saving treatment available. In haemolytic disease of the newborn it is the only treatment available. As already stated, single unit transfusions are rarely justifiable, although it should be noted that a case can be made out for them in some circumstances.[14] In countries where patients are required to pay for the blood they receive there is the risk that small-volume transfusions may be given for financial rather than medical reasons.

The risks of transfusion are many. Chance bacterial contamination, transmission of disease, blood group incompatibility and the risks of blood group immunisation, are especially important. Blood is not a magic substance and the advantages to the patient in terms of his condition (and not merely his convenience) should be carefully balanced against the risks. So called 'cosmetic' transfusions, given for no scientifically supportable reason, are inexcusable. In Great Britain the abuse of blood transfusion is minimal; in other countries — particularly the U.S.A. — there is evidence that this is not always so.[14, 15] Nevertheless, the fact that the practice of blood transfusion can be abused does not *ipso facto* make the practice as such undesirable, as the Jehovah's Witnesses suggest.[2]

REFERENCES

[1] Mollison, P. L. (1967), *Blood Transfusion in Clinical Medicine* (4th edn.). Blackwell, London.

[2] *Blood, Medicine, and the Law of God* (1961). Watch Tower Bible and Tract Society, New York.

[3] Coventry & Dis' Voluntary Blood Donors' Ass'n Newsletter. 34th edn. Feb. 1963).

[4] British Pharmacopoeia. 1963. Pharmaceutical Press, London.

[5] National Research Council (1951), *Decompression Sickness*. p. 49. W. B. Saunders, Philadelphia and London.

[6] Race, R. R., and Sanger, R. (1968), *Blood Groups in Man* (5th edn.) Blackwell, London.

[7] Farr, A. D. (1963), *A Synopsis of Blood Group Theory and Serological Techniques*. Heinemann, London.

[8] *The Separation of Protein Fractions from Human Plasma with Ether*. M.R.C. Special Report Series No. 286. H.M.S.O., London.

[9] Grünbaum, A. S., and Grünbaum, H. G. (1911), *B.M.Jnl. ii,* 1281.

[10] See references in 1. pp. 109-111.

[11] Ebert, R. V., Stead, E. A., and Gibson, J. G. (1941), *Arch Intern. Med. 68*. 578.

[12] Wadsworth, G. R. (1955). *J. Physiol.* (Lond). *129,* 583.

[13] Crosby, W. H. (1958) *M. Bull. U.S. Army, Europe. 15,* 3.

[14] Crosby, W. H. (1964), *Transfusion, 4,* 329.

[15] Pirofsky, B. (1960), *G.P.* (September. 128.

[16] Discombe, G. (1955), *Blood Transfusion*. Heinemann, London.

3

JEHOVAH'S WITNESSES

'We are an anachronism. We are living at a time when religious belief is a triviality to most people, but to us it is the most important thing in the world. We believe the Bible — quite literally. We don't just pay lip service to it, but try to live everything it says, and this brings us into conflict with many people. Our belief that we should not accept blood transfusions is based on what the Bible says.'

This description was given by Mr. Wilfred Gooch, described as 'leader of the Witnesses in Britain', in an article in *World Medicine* on 12 November 1968, and it is not an unreasonable brief summary.

The Watch Tower Bible and Tract Society is the present organisation of the church founded by Charles Taze Russell. Russell was born in the United States of America in 1852 and died in 1916. It is said that Russell as a child received a strong impression of the terrors of hell from the Congregational church which the family attended. His fears were set at rest by an atheist whom he met, but it is a significant fact that the movement which he later founded preaches the non-existence of hell. While there can be no pleasure in considering evidence damaging to the character of an individual now dead, it would be unrealistic to ignore certain facts concerning Russell, particularly where these bear on the question of Bible translation which may seriously affect interpretation. Russell was frequently involved in law-suits (including his own divorce proceedings in which he received some unfavourable publicity) and in one of these he affirmed under oath that he knew Greek. It was easily demonstrated with the aid of a Greek New Testament that this was not true, and under cross-examination he admitted to having no knowledge of Greek, Latin or Hebrew. One of Russell's main contentions, still followed by Jehovah's Witnesses, is that all Bible translations (other than that now published by the Watch Tower Society) are unsatisfactory and all other churches anti-Christian.

In 1872 at Allegheny near Pittsburgh, Pennsylvania, Russell started a Bible class that came together regularly with the object of studying the scriptures about Jehovah's kingdom and the second coming of Christ Jesus. Soon, similar groups were organized throughout the United States, and later on they spread to other countries. The printed courses of scripture studies used by the groups were offered from door to door by members, and this method of preaching has remained the way used to spread the teaching of the Society. In 1916, following Russell's death, the leadership of the organisation was taken over by 'Judge' J. F. Rutherford.

Rutherford was born in 1869 and was granted a licence to practice law in 1892, although he was never in fact a judge. Following Russell's death Rutherford served nine months in gaol for seditious utterances. This was regarded by adherents of the faith as persecution and served to enhance his reputation. He died in 1942 at the age of seventy-two. The sect is now controlled by Nathan H. Knorr.

Various names have been used by the followers of Russell. For many years they were known as 'Bible

Students' or 'International Bible Students', but at a convention held at Columbus, Ohio, in 1931 the name 'Jehovah's Witnesses' was agreed upon and has been used ever since. ('Ye are my witnesses, saith Jehovah.' Is. 43: 10, 44: 8.) In 1884 the body of the International Bible Students was incorporated under Pennsylvania law as the Watch Tower Bible and Tract Society, and the headquarters moved in 1909 from Pittsburgh to New York. This Society, under other names in some countries, continues today as the legal governing body of Jehovah's Witnesses. At various times members of the society have also been called Russellites, Millennial Dawnites, Rutherfordites, the Metropolitan Pulpit, and Brooklyn Tabernacle Pulpit.

Jehovah's Witnesses do not have salaried ministers, each witness being bound to give his own testimony and pay his own expenses. Although there is no formal course of training leading to ordination, ministers of the society claim and receive, in Britain and the U.S.A., at least, exemption from military service. Jehovah's Witnesses claim to be 'a society of ministers . . . a group of evangelists, all being ministers, just as those in the first congregation of Christ Jesus were ministers, each and all. Each active minister has as his congregation a group of people of good will to whom he ministers at their homes in territory assigned to him. Such a minister goes to the people. They do not have to seek him out to learn about God's kingdom'. (LGT. pp. 224-225)

The belief of Jehovah's Witnesses centre upon their conviction that the Bible is the inspired word of God and, as such, is to be read and interpreted literally. They reject utterly the use of oral tradition. The stand taken is that as the Bible is the word of God, it is not open to interpretation in the light of tradition or experience as this would imply that ' the Bible's Author was all mixed up and divided against himself ' (LGT. p. 8). Consequently the Bible is to be read and studied as literal truth. ' Let God be found true, though every man be found a liar.' (Romans 3: 4). This first assumption accounts for nearly all the beliefs of Jehovah's Witnesses which differ from those of orthodox Christianity, where it is recognised that great truths expressed in the Bible may be presented in the form of allegory or parable and, in places, symbolically.

The Witnesses believe that only God the Father — whom they call Jehovah — is almighty. His son Jesus Christ is neither eternal nor God, but a created being who is regarded like an archangel (NHNE. pp. 26-28). ' The relationship of the Father and Son may be compared to a business where there is a President and under him an executive who carries out the wishes of the President ' (Look, p. 13). The Holy Spirit is an impersonal ' active force of Almighty God ' (LGT. p. 108). The doctrine of a Holy Trinity is entirely rejected as being ' a complicated, freakish-looking, three-headed God ' (LGT. p. 102). Jehovah's Witnesses are thus seen not to be Christians, as they claim, but while monotheistic in outlook, they are frankly unitarian.

Jesus' death is seen as a ransom not for the sins of mankind but for the perfect human life which Adam lost for himself and his offspring by his sinning; the gift of Jesus' life, a perfect man created by God, in exchange for the perfect life which Adam was originally given. By His death on the cross Jesus obtained not ' everlasting life to any man, but only a second chance ' (Truth Shall . . . p. 177). The resurrection of Christ is seen as the raising of a spirit creature (GNK p. 14) and the bodily resurrection is denied.

Jehovah's Witnesses deny that there is an afterlife for mankind in heaven or hell. They teach that Christ's second coming occurred in 1874 as an invisible event and that in 1914 He took up His kingdom power in heaven, where He will be joined by 144,000 elect, who will help Him to rule over mankind. These 144,000 have been selected by Christ gradually since His life here on earth, and a small remnant of them are still with us amongst Jehovah's Witnesses. On taking up His kingdom Christ forced the Devil out of the heavens, and his return to earth was signalled (with the World War) by the onset of tribulation forecast in Matthew 24: 7-8 (' Nation shall rise against nation, and kingdom against kingdom: and there shall be famines, and pestilences, and earthquakes in divers places. All these are the beginning of sorrows.'). In the course of time, Jesus and His angels will have a final battle with Satan, called Armageddon, and all ' the invisible and visible parts of Satan's world ' will be destroyed (LGT. p. 259). Following Armageddon the earthly survivors will live and procreate, together with 'millions of "unrighteous" dead ' (LGT p. 270) who will be resurrected and taught the truth about Jehovah, and for 1,000 years Christ will reign over the earth with His heavenly ' parliament ' of 144,000 while there is perfect peace and concord. After the millenium the Devil and his demons will be released from the pit to try to overthrow Jehovah's kingdom, and eventually will be thrown, with his followers, into everlasting destruction. There will then be no more procreation of children, but love and peace on earth for ever.

Jehovah's Witnesses are amongst the bodies which practise baptism by total immersion and they believe that even those previously baptised must be baptised again into their faith. They regard the orthodox Christian churches as the agents of the Devil, particularly in view of their support of the ideals of the United Nations, which organisation they identify with 'the scarlet-colored, seven-headed, ten-horned, wild beast ascended out of the abyss,' referred to in Revelation 17: 3 and 17: 8 (NHNE, p. 279). The Witnesses claim allegiance only to Jehovah's Kingdom, and refuse to give homage to the flag of any earthly nation. They deplore patriotism and this attitude has led to considerable persecution and/or proscription in many countries, including, at various times, Northern and Southern Rhodesia, New Zealand, Australia, Nazi Germany, all the communist countries and many independent African states (the latest of which are Tanzania and Cameroon). In 1947 the Supreme Court of Canada ruled that they were 'not a religious body'. In Portugal recently a number of Witnesses have been arraigned on a charge of belonging to a religious group whose ideas 'are contrary to the present political situation'.

As will be seen from the foregoing, Jehovah's Witnesses take their stand upon very literal interpretations of the Bible and, indeed, in some cases their own translation is phrased so as to provide an entirely different interpretation from that generally accepted. A classic example of this is found in Luke 23: 43 where Jesus comforts the penitent thief on the cross. The Authorised Version reads 'Verily I say unto thee, Today thou shall be with me in paradise'. Jehovah's Witnesses do not accept the after-life of the spirit and by the simple movement of a comma cause their New World translation to read 'Truly I tell you today, You will be with me in paradise' *in the far distant future* (NHNE, p. 349). Such highly interpreted readings of the scriptures and manipulations in translation will be seen much in evidence in considering their attitude to blood transfusion in the next chapter.

REFERENCES

<table>
<tr><td>LGT</td><td>Let God be True (2nd edn.)</td><td rowspan="5">Watch Tower Bible and Tract Society, New York and London</td></tr>
<tr><td>NHNE</td><td>New Heavens and a New Earth</td></tr>
<tr><td>GNK</td><td>Good News of the Kingdom</td></tr>
<tr><td>Look</td><td>Look, I make all things new</td></tr>
<tr><td></td><td>New World Translation of the Holy Scriptures (Revised 2nd edn.)</td></tr>
</table>

Commentaries

Some Modern Religions: Sanders, J. O. and Wright, J. S. (4th edn.) (1963), Tyndale Press, London.

Jehovah's Witnesses: Church Book Room Press, London

Sects and Society: Wilson, B. R. (1961), Heinemann, London.

Christian Deviations: The Challenge of the Sects: Davies, H. (1954), SCM, London.

4

THE THEOLOGICAL ARGUMENTS

MOST of the more than four hundred references to blood in the Bible can be divided into four main groups: those referring to blood shed by violence; the blood of Christ; blood used for sacrificial purposes; and prohibitions on the eating of blood. It is these last two groups that are used by Jehovah's Witnesses as authority for their rejection of blood transfusion.

It is necessary to recall at this point the stand taken by Jehovah's Witnesses on the literal truth of the Bible. They say that the Bible is the only guide to the truth '. . . accept His Word, the Bible, as the truth' (LGT, p. 9). They claim that the Bible *in toto* is the inspired word of God. 'Knowing that God by His holy spirit inspired the Holy Scriptures, thus making them reliable, we choose to let Him do the interpreting' (LGT, pp. 18-19). Thus they claim that the Bible is capable of only one interpretation at any point. 'Reasonably, then, His Book, the Bible, could not be all mixed up and allowing any interpretation to be made of it' (LGT, p. 8). Their position is stated clearly in another book. 'For the good of the generations to come He *(God)* has turned Author and has caused this revelation to be written under inspiration in the Holy Scriptures' (NHNE, p. 17). Now while admitting that much of the Bible consists of the inspired word of God, one must accept that it was written down by the hand of fallible man, and that in the process some of man's fallibility became written-in also. By what other explanation can one understand the many instances of contradiction to be found, particularly in the Old Testament? Two examples from each Testament of these contradictions are given below as examples.

OLD TESTAMENT

The creation of man:
- On the sixth day (Gen. 1: 27)
- After the seventh day (Gen. 2: 7)

The creation of woman:
- At the same time as Adam (Gen. 1: 27)
- From Adam's rib (Gen. 2: 21-22)

NEW TESTAMENT

Finding the empty tomb:
- Two Marys find an angel outside (Matt. 28: 1-7)
- Two Marys and Salome find a young man inside (Mark 16: 1-5)
- Mary Magdalene, Peter and John. Mary sees two angels (John 20: 1-13)

First resurrection:
- In Galilee, to the eleven disciples (Matt. 28: 16-17)
- At Emmaus (near Jerusalem) to two disciples (Luke 24: 13-31)
- At the tomb to Mary Magdalene (John 20: 14-17), and in Jerusalem to all the disciples (John 20: 19-29)

There are perfectly adequate explanations for the multiplicity of accounts of various incidents throughout the Bible, but amongst these is not the Jehovah's Witnesses' suggestion 'that the Bible's Author was all mixed up and divided against himself' (LGT, p. 8), with which statement they dismiss the possibility of the Bible being anywhere subject to interpretation. To allege that every word, every phrase in the Bible was directly 'dictated' by God to the various writers would to be to deprive man of free-will. Even the Witnesses do not suggest that man is subject to predestination. Indeed they state categorically of God, '. . . He did not choose to predestinate the individuals . . .' (NHNE, p. 159). This same argument of free will is, indeed, generally accepted to refute the legend that the septuagint of the Hebrew scriptures into Greek was made in 70 identical versions, completed simultaneously, by 70 scribes. Paul in his epistle to the Galatians warned the church of attempts to pervert its teaching, and the words are as pertinent to the Christian church today, with its received teaching of nearly 2,000 years which, especially on the point of the Mosaic Law, has never been in dispute. 'As we have said before, so say I now again, If any man preacheth unto you any gospel other than that which ye received, let him be anathema' Gal. 1: 9. R.V.).

The Christian church has always used the Bible as a guide to God's will rather than as a text book of ritual observance. There is no evidence to suggest that this is not still the right course.

With the Witnesses' attitude in mind one may now study the relevant texts (given here in the Authorized Version).

After the deluge God gave to Noah the instruction, 'Every moving thing that liveth shall be meat for you;

even as the green herb have I given you all things. But flesh with the life thereof, which is the blood thereof, shall ye not eat' (Genesis 9: 3-4). In the book of Leviticus, where the priestly law was given by God to Moses this prohibition on the eating of blood was repeated several times. 'It shall be a perpetual statute for your generations throughout all your dwellings, that ye eat neither fat nor blood' (Lev. 3: 17). 'Moreover ye shall eat no manner of blood whether it be of fowl or of beast, in any of your dwellings. Whatsoever soul it be that eateth any manner of blood, even that soul shall be cut off from his people' (Lev. 7: 26-27). 'And whatsoever man there be of the house of Israel, or of the strangers that sojourn among you, that eateth any manner of blood, I will even set my face against that soul that eateth blood, and will cut him off from among his people. For the life of the flesh is in the blood: and I have given it to you upon the altar to make an atonement for the soul. Therefore I said unto the children of Israel, No soul of you shall eat blood, neither shall any stranger that sojourneth among you eat blood. And whatsoever man there be of the children of Israel, or of the strangers that sojourn among you, which hunteth and catcheth any beast or fowl that may be eaten; he shall even pour out the blood thereof, and cover it with dust. For it is the life of all flesh; the blood of it is for the life thereof: therefore I said unto the children of Israel, Ye shall eat the blood of no manner of flesh: for the life of all flesh is the blood thereof: whosoever eateth it shall be cut off' (Lev. 17: 10-14). 'Ye shall not eat anything with the blood: neither shall ye use enchantment, nor observe times' (Lev. 19: 26). In the book of Deuteronomy Moses repeats to a new generation of the Israelites the basis of the covenant. (It is noteworthy that parts of Deuteronomy abrogate some of the law given in Leviticus, and replace it, thus indicating that the earlier law is not immutable. (For example, see Deut. 12: 15 and Lev. 17: 3-5). The law about eating blood is again repeated. 'Only ye shall not eat the blood; ye shall pour it upon the earth as water' (Deut. 12: 16). 'Even as the roebuck and the hart is eaten, so thou shalt eat them: the unclean and the clean eat of them alike. Only be sure that thou eat not the blood; for the blood is the life; and thou mayest not eat the life with the flesh. Thou shalt not eat it; thou shalt pour it upon the earth as water' (Deut. 12: 22-24).

The New Testament contains only two (related) direct references to the eating of blood. In AD 52 the church at Jerusalem was considering the application of circumcision and other ritual aspects of Judaism to the gentile converts to Christianity. St. James suggested '. . . that we write unto them, that they abstain from pollution of idols, and from fornication, and from things strangled, and from blood' (Acts 15: 20). The actual letter written to the church at Antioch said — amongst other things — 'That ye abstain from meats offered to idols, and from blood and from things strangled, and from fornication: from which, if ye keep yourselves, ye shall do well' (Acts 15: 29).

It will be noted that all of the Old Testament references given refer specifically to the eating of blood. The two references in Acts require separate consideration and will be dealt with accordingly.

Study of the references will be directed to four aspects. Firstly applicability of these Jewish laws to the Christian church, secondly the type of blood referred to, thirdly the reasons for the prohibition, and finally the relationship between eating and blood transfusion which is alleged by Jehovah's Witnesses. In each case various translations of the scriptures will be considered.

The laws given to Moses under the covenant were given not to mankind as a whole, but to the people of Israel — God's chosen people — and included in a codified form much that had been given to God's people on previous occasions, such as the prohibition on eating blood given to Noah (Gen. 9: 3-4).

'And the Lord called unto Moses, and spake unto him out of the tabernacle of the congregation, saying, Speak unto the children of Israel, and say unto them, . . .' (Lev. 1: 1-2). And again: 'And the Lord spake unto Moses, saying, Speak unto Aaron, and unto his sons, and unto all the children of Israel, and say unto them; This is the thing which the Lord hath commanded, saying,' (Lev. 17: 1-2): 'And the Lord spake unto Moses, saying, Speak unto all the congregation of the children of Israel and say unto them, . . .' (Lev. 19: 1-2). In Deuteronomy the repeated prohibitions are prefaced, 'Hear, O Israel . . .' (Deut. 9: 1). It seems abundantly clear therefore that the laws of the covenant were addressed in the first place to the people of Israel. It is moeover clear from Lev. 17: 10 and 17: 12-13 that the prohibition extended to 'the strangers that sojourn among you'. In their New World translation the expression used by Jehovah's Witnesses is 'alien resident who is residing as an alien in your midst'. Whatever the merits of this as a translation it would certainly seem in this case to be at least a good transliteration. We might express it today as 'when in Rome, do as the

Romans do '. The extension of the prohibition is merely to other peoples living amongst the Israelites.

It is true that Lev. 7: 27 says '*Whatsoever soul* it be that eateth any manner of blood, even that soul shall be cut off from his people ' and again in Lev. 17: 14 '. . . *whosoever* eateth it shall be cut off '. It seems obvious that as these references are in the context of a law delivered specifically to the Israelites — a people who believed that they alone were God's people — they refer only to those people, and not to the gentiles. The Witnesses would believe otherwise, taking the phrases out of their context and reading them literally as applying to all mankind.

Having established that the law regarding blood was in the first instance given solely to the people of Israel, it is necessary to consider to what extent the law may be applicable to the Christian church which sprang out of Judaism, which continues to worship the same one God, and which is almost exclusively gentile.

Jesus said, 'Think not that I am come to destroy the law, or the prophets; I am come not to destroy, but to fulfil ' (Matt. 5: 17). This was of course spoken by a Jew to a Jewish audience. Subsequently our Lord showed that by ' fulfilment ' He meant amplification and reasonable application of the law (e.g. the plucking of corn on the Sabbath. Matt. 12: 1-6). He also said after His resurrection ' . . . thus it behoved Christ to suffer, and to rise from the dead the third day, And that repentance and remission of sins should be preached in His name among all nations, . . . ' (Luke 24: 46-47). The commission was clearly to preach repentance and remission in Christ's name — not Jewish law. On the night of the last supper Jesus confirmed that He was come to make a *new* covenant between God and man (' For this is my blood of the new testament, which is shed for many for the remission of sins ' (Matt. 26: 28)). The principles of the new covenant were broadly based upon those of the old, but one of the effects of Christ's coming was to free men of the tedious and rigid adherence to the letter of the law, while stressing more the spirit of it. ' Christ hath redeemed us from the curse of the law, . . . ' (Gal. 3: 13). ' For the law made nothing perfect, but the bringing in of a better hope did; by the which we draw nigh unto God ' (Heb. 7: 19). Knowing that a man is not justified by the works of the law, but by the faith of Jesus Christ, even we have believed in Jesus Christ, that we might be justified by the faith of Christ, and not by the works of the law: for by the works of the law shall no flesh be justified ' (Gal. 2: 16). ' For the law was given by Moses, but grace and truth came by Jesus Christ ' (John 1: 17). St. Paul, writing to the church at Collossae, spelled the effects of this out in no uncertain terms. ' Let no man therefore judge you in meat, or in drink, or in respect of an holyday, or of the new moon, or of the sabbath days: which are a shadow of things to come; but the body is of Christ ' (Collossians 2: 16-17). This conforms with St. Peter's speech before the assembly in Jerusalem in 52AD, when he said (God) ' . . . put no difference between us and them, purifying their hearts by faith. Now wherefore why tempt ye God, to put a yoke upon the neck of the disciples, which neither our fathers nor we were able to bear? ' (Acts. 15: 9-10). Clearly the rigid observance of the Jewish law was not binding upon the new Christian church.

The two references in Acts (Ch. 15 vv. 20 and 29) can

be a source of some difficulty, and indeed are the sole positive biblical bases of argument used by the Witnesses for their application of the law regarding blood to Christians. In order to understand these it is necessary to look at the verses, not standing on their own, but in the context of the whole 15th chapter. The gentile church at Antioch was perplexed by certain teachers who claimed that it was necessary for converts to be circumcised according to Jewish law, thus raising again an issue which had already been settled fifteen years previously in the case of the centurion Cornelius (Acts 10: 1-48). The matter was brought before the assembly of the church at Jerusalem (Acts 15: 4-12), who reached the decision that gentile converts need not be circumcised. (' . . . that we should impose no irksome restrictions on those of the Gentiles who are turning to God ' (Acts 15: 19 NEB)) thus formally acknowledging the truly universal nature of the church. It was, however, decided to write to the church at Antioch to ' . . . instruct them by letter to abstain from things polluted by contact with idols, from fornication, from anything that has been strangled, and from blood ' (Acts 15: 20 NEB). The reason for this is clearly stated in the next verse — and perhaps most clearly so in the Jehovah's Witnesses' own translation. ' For from ancient times Moses has had in city after city those who preach him, because he is read aloud in the synagogues on every sabbath ' (Acts 15: 21 NW). In other words, the gentile converts are being warned against some of the usages forbidden in the Mosaic Law, thus being taught consideration for the Jews, who were still taught the obligations of that Law. At this time the Christian church at Antioch was the only established gentile church in an otherwise entirely Jewish faith; the '. . . alien in your midst . . .' envisaged in Leviticus (Ch. 17 v. 10. NW). It is noticeable that this warning is addressed solely to the church at Antioch at that time. On later occasions when the number of gentile churches had greatly increased we find repetitions of the warnings against the practices tending to idolatry (e.g. 1 Cor. 8 *and* 10) and against immorality (e.g. 1 Cor. 5: 9) but nowhere else is there a repetition of the warning against blood. The inescapable conclusion is that this warning, as was the Mosaic Law before it, was directed solely to one group of people, and for reasons connected solely with the stage of development of the Christian church at that early time. Had it been otherwise it is hard to see why St. Paul did not mention this point along with the others which he did repeat for the benefit of other churches, or why it was not mentioned again in other letters which went to the churches in Syria (the general epistles of St. James, St. Peter and St. John). It is true that for many years Christians did respect the Jewish law with regard to the eating of blood and of things strangled, but this was a self-imposed discipline which soon died out.

Despite the evidence adduced to relate the Mosaic Law solely to the Jews, Jehovah's Witnesses continue to maintain that the prohibition on blood applies to all men for all time (*Blood, Medicine and the Law of God,* pp. 6-10). This is totally illogical in view of their assertions, laid out in full in Chapter XVI of *Let God be True,* that the Mosaic Law was abolished *in toto* by Christ's *new* covenant. They state categorically '. . . that such Law was abolished and brought to an end by Jehovah, and that no creatures on earth, not even the

Jews, are any longer under it' (LGT, p. 183). The Witnesses' literature on the application of the Law to Christians is indeed a tangled and tortuous path to travel. In the book *Blood, Medicine and the Law of God,* they quote authorities to claim that this part of the Law has alone never been revoked (p. 6) — yet in *Let God be True* they say 'The law covenant cannot be taken apart, so that a part of it . . . could be abolished . . .' (LGT, p. 188). They go on to remind us indeed of St. James's words, 'For if a man keeps the whole law apart from one single point, he is guilty of breaking all of it' (James 2: 10 NEB), while at the same time admitting that the Mosaic Law no longer applies to Christians. One cannot have it both ways. If the Law does not apply to Christians, the Christian church cannot remain bound to just one single provision of it.

It may appear superfluous to consider what sort of blood is referred to in the Mosaic Laws, but there are in fact two reasons for so doing. Firstly, there is not one single reference in the Bible to the eating of human blood and, secondly, there comes a point at which it is necessary to define what we mean by the word 'blood'.

All of the ten Old Testament references to eating blood are included in ordinances referring to food (Gen. 9: 4, Lev. 3: 17, 7: 26: 27; 17: 10, 12: 14, 19: 26, Deut. 12: 16: 23). The Witnesses do not deny this, nor that the eating of human blood is nowhere specifically mentioned. They take their stand on the wording of the texts which refer to '. . . any manner of blood . . .' (Lev. 7: 27, 17: 10). Now if one thing is certain, it is that the Jewish people have never at any time in their history practised cannibalism, despite the wording of

Genesis 9: 3-4, which says 'Every moving thing that liveth shall be meat for you; even as the green herb have I given you all things'. If one accepts the absolute literal truth of the Bible one must agree that this ruling implicitly allows the eating of human flesh, especially as nowhere in the Bible is this directly forbidden. Yet the Witnesses would not normally dream of practising cannibalism, any more than have the Jews. Neither have the Jews ever used any form of ritual which requires the drinking (or eating) of the blood of one another or of their victims in battle. Such acts were indulged in by some ancient peoples (see Tertullian's *Apology,* also Psalm 16: 4) but at no point in history have the Jews ever been accused of the practice. It is abundantly clear that the wording used by the (human and, therefore, fallible) scribes who recorded these things was intended to apply solely to that which was known to, and readily accessible to, the Jews of that time; that is the blood of the animals and fowl used by them for food. There is not even any suggestion in Jewish history of its application to insects (such as locusts) which were sometimes used for food, and which also contain blood. To suggest that laws relating to animals used for food also extend to human blood is to start placing unwarranted interpretations on the Bible, a practice which they themselves thoroughly deplore (*Let God be True,* Chap. I). By making such assumptions the Witnesses ignore their own exhortation, 'To arrive at truth we must dismiss religious prejudices from heart and mind. We must let God speak for Himself' (LGT, p. 8).

To consider what we mean by 'blood' is not as simple a matter as may at first appear. To the people of Israel blood was doubtless a simple fluid found in the body. Even today it is no more to most people. *The Shorter Oxford English Dictionary* defines blood as: 'The red liquid circulating in the arteries and veins of man and the higher animals'. There is no doubt that at the time the Law was given 'blood' would mean exactly that — the red liquid. How then do the Witnesses base their refusal to accept blood components such as plasma, which is a light golden yellow colour, or fibrinogen which is white? They claim that '. . . it is not just whole blood but anything that is derived from blood . . . that comes under this principle' (*Watchtower,* Feb. 15, 1963). Here again, however, they are bending the words of the Bible to achieve their own meaning, in defiance of their own objections to such behaviour already mentioned. The Bible does not forbid albumin, globulins, or any other component of blood, it refers simply to *blood* and means just that, i.e. the whole blood. In this connection a further inconsistency may be found in Jehovah's Witness theology. Despite the firm line taken on the principle of refusing any part of blood, they allow their members the freedom of their own conscience as to whether or not they accept prophylactic anti-sera, which are pure animal serum (i.e. the fluid portion of blood which has been allowed to clot and which is similar to plasma). In an authoritative ruling on this point in the *Watchtower* of September 15, 1958 (p. 575) it is stated, 'It would, therefore, be a matter of individual judgment whether one accepted such types of medication or not'. The ruling claims that this particular use of blood is objectionable but not forbidden. They allow indeed the pressures of society to determine the matter '. . . vaccination is a virtually unavoidable practice in many segments of modern society . . .' (*Watchtower*, November 1, 1961, p. 669). A viewpoint which contrasts strangely with the question and answer in *Awake!* (January 22, 1958, p. 22). 'Would you rather die than take blood? Yes. I do not want to die but I cannot place even my own life above God's law.' It would seem that the theology of the Witnesses on the point of blood components is inconsistent. If they may receive serum from animals, the blood of which is mentioned in Mosaic Law, why may they not receive serum (or plasma) from a human source when human blood is not mentioned?

It is relevant to this discussion to consider the reasons behind the prohibitions on blood contained in Jewish Law. Quite apart from any religious explanation, the draining of blood from freshly killed animals intended to be used as food was a perfectly sound practice on grounds of pure hygiene. At the time the Mosaic Law was given the people of Israel were entering the second year of their wanderings following the exodus from Egypt. The wilderness in the Sinai Peninsula (present day Saudi-Arabia) is one of the hottest areas in the world and meat drained of blood would be less susceptible to spoilage and deterioration in such a climate than would that which was not drained. Such considerations are, however, pure speculation. The reasons given in the Bible are entirely religious.

The basic reason for prohibiting the eating of blood is given in Leviticus 17: 11, 'For the life of the flesh is in the blood: and I have given it to you upon the altar to make an atonement for your souls: for it is the blood that maketh an atonement for the soul'. The Revised Version translates the last phrase 'for it is the blood that maketh atonement by reason of the life'. The Jehovah's Witness New World translation renders the verse in yet another way, 'For the soul of the flesh is in the blood, and I myself have put it upon the altar for you to make atonement for your souls, because it is the blood that makes atonement by the soul of it'. This divergent reading is repeated in verse 14, where the A.V. and R.V. say, 'for the life of all flesh is the blood thereof'. The New World translation of this passage reads 'because the soul of every sort of flesh is its blood'. In Deuteronomy, where the reference is directly to the roebuck and the hart (the gazelle and the stag N.W.) as sources of food we read, 'Only be sure that thou eat not the blood: for the blood is the life; and thou mayest not eat the life with the flesh' (Deut. 12: 23). Here again the New World translation differs. 'Simply be firmly resolved not to eat the blood, because the blood is the soul and you must not eat the soul with the flesh'. The New World Translation Committee explain in their translation (Revised Edition, 1961, p. 1445) that they have consistently rendered the Hebrew *neph'esh* (Greek, psy-khē) as 'soul' despite its appearance in many different contexts. This is in contrast with other translators who have taken context into account and rendered the word as either 'soul' or 'life'. This latter course is the one taken by the New English Bible Committee in their New Testament translation also published in 1961. Whatever the merits or otherwise of the New English Bible as literature, it is universally accepted as the most definitive translation yet produced, and is based upon the best manuscripts available and the latest advances in knowledge of the everyday Greek of the first century. In the light of this the consistent translation of *neph'esh* and *psy-khē* as 'soul' in the New World version would appear to be unjustified.

Whether the blood is to be regarded as the life or as the soul of an animal, the real reason for it being prohibited as food is clearly given by God: '... I myself have put it upon the altar for you to make atonement for your souls ...' (Lev. 17: 11 NW). In other words, blood was reserved by God for sacrificial purposes. It was not to be profaned by secular use. Blood not used on the altar for sacrifice was to be spilled on the ground: '... pour out the blood thereof, and cover it with dust' (Lev. 17: 13), '... ye shall pour it upon the earth as water' (Deut. 12: 16, 24). The sacrificial uses of blood are amply documented (Ex. 23: 18, 24: 6: 8; Lev. 1: 5, 3: 2: 8: 13, 4: 5-7: 16-18, 5: 9, 17: 6). In the light of this, one would feel that consistent theology would demand that blood be put to no purpose whatever other than sacrificial. The Witnesses themselves state: 'They are not going to feel that if they have some of their own blood stored for transfusion, it is going to be more acceptable than the blood of another person. They know that God required that shed blood be poured out on the ground. Nor are they going to feel that a slight infraction, such as momentary storage of blood in a syringe when it is drawn from one part of the body for injection into another part, is somehow less objectionable than storing it for a longer period of time. They are not trying to see how close they can walk to the line without overstepping the Law' (*Blood, Medicine and the Law of God,* pp. 14-15). In the light of these lofty sentiments one wonders at the acceptance by Jehovah's Witnesses of open heart surgery involving a heart-lung machine of the 'Miniprime' type. In this procedure the machine is initially filled with a solution of dextrose, and then connected at two points with the patient's circulation. The patient's blood passes continuously through the machine, in which it is oxygenated and pumped back into the body, by-passing the heart and lungs and thus enabling major surgery to be performed on these organs. This procedure for eliminating donor blood may be more hazardous than when such blood is used, but was developed into a technique suitable for use on Jehovah's Witness patients. So important is this application felt to be that the American manufacturers of the apparatus (Baxter Laboratories) have produced a teaching film *Open heart surgery in a Jehovah's Witness* in which the procedure is demonstrated and two Witnesses who have benefited by the operation are shown during surgery and after recovery. This procedure involves considerably more than 'momentary storage of blood in a syringe', yet it appears to be acceptable. An article 'Surgery without Blood Transfusions' in *Awake!* for July 22, 1965, confirms this. Again we are faced with an inconsistency in Witness teaching. It may also be pointed out here that even the orthodox Jews of the 20th century have never objected to the practice of blood transfusion upon these grounds, nor to any other medical procedure in which blood is taken from a patient for investigation. There are indeed Jehovah's Witnesses practising as nurses, doctors, even pathologists, who are inevitably required to collect and test such blood samples. The fact that the bulk of their patients are not Witnesses is immaterial, as they relate the prohibition on secular use of blood to animal blood even, let alone that of other humans. Again, in an article entitled 'Carry your own load of responsibilities' (*Watchtower,* Feb. 15, 1963) it is made clear that it is a matter of conscience to the individual whether or not he takes part in secular activities in which blood is used. In 'Employment and your conscience' (*Watchtower,* Nov. 15, 1964) a long list is given of things encountered in every day life in which products of animal blood may be met, including a great many items which are made with certain adhesives. In connection with these the advice is given '. . . the Christian is not responsible for the worldly misuse of blood'. A strange attitude in the light of Christ's admonition, '. . . Thou shalt love thy neighbour as thyself' (Matt. 22: 39). In the same article the matter is clearly left open. 'Because blood may be used in some plywood, this does not mean that a Christian could not buy, sell or rent a home or purchase a trailer in which plywood is found.' And again, '. . . if a Christian is working for a company that uses blood glue in some of its plywood or other products, he would not necessarily have to quit his job'. Yet the official Jehovah's Witness instruction is, 'Keep yourselves free . . . from blood' (Acts 15: 29 NW); '. . . any sort of blood . . .' (Lev. 17: 10 NW). We would appear to be faced again with the wish to have things both ways.

Possibly the most difficult thing for the orthodox Christian to understand about Jehovah's Witnesses' attitude towards blood transfusion is how they relate the eating of blood to blood transfusion. Every one of the Old Testament prohibitions on blood refers specifically to the eating of blood. *The Shorter Oxford English Dictionary* defines *eat* thus: 'Masticate and swallow as food. To feed destructively upon'. This definition is exactly that which is understood by most people.

The act of eating leads to a well defined metabolic process. The food is acted upon by various chemicals within the body, during the process of which action it is entirely broken up and converted into a form in which it can be absorbed into the body, with the exception of a certain bulk which, after the extraction of all that the body can use, is excreted. The process is entirely destructive as regards the food itself. The useful parts of the food are converted into material used for making new tissue, stores of fat, etc., and into energy. This is the process called metabolism.

On the other hand the process of blood transfusion consists of the introduction into the circulation of an additional quantity of ready-formed blood. The transfused blood mixes with that of the patient and supplements it, without being in any way altered itself. The various constituents of blood all have a limited life, and as each constituent reaches the end of its life it is eliminated from the circulation. The process takes place both in the case of a patient's own blood and of any transfused blood in his circulation. The handling involved in collection and storage do, it is true, reduce the post-transfusion survival time of certain blood components slightly. The unaltered transfused blood is not converted by the recipient's body into anything — it merely continues its main function of gas transport.

The attitude of Jehovah's Witnesses is '. . . that by a direct route the blood serves the same purpose as food when taken into the stomach, namely, strengthening the body or sustaining life' (*Watchtower,* Feb. 15, 1963); '. . . a transfusion is practically the same as intravenous feeding. The fact that in blood transfusion the blood is merely being replaced makes no difference. The only other way this can be done is by foods that will build more blood. A transfusion is just a more direct way of accomplishing this result' (*Awake!*, Jan. 22, 1958). 'It has no bearing on the matter that the blood is not introduced to the body through the mouth but through the veins. Nor does the argument that it cannot be classed with intravenous feeding because its use in the body is different carry weight. The fact is that it provides nourishment to the body to sustain life' (*Blood, Medicine and the Law of God*, p. 14). In support of these contentions, this latter booklet quotes Denys, a French physician and transfusionist, as saying: 'In performing transfusion it is nothing else than nourishing by a shorter road than ordinary — that is to say, placing in the veins blood all made in place of taking food which only turns to blood after several changes' (p. 14). They omit to mention that Denys performed his first transfusion experiments in 1667, only thirty-nine years after Harvey published his discovery that blood circulated around the body. Their position is clearly summed up thus: '. . . regardless of the method used to infuse it into the body and regardless of whether it is whole blood or a blood substance that is involved, God's law remains the same. If it is blood and it is being used to nourish or to sustain life the divine law clearly applies' (*Blood, Medicine and the Law of God*, p. 14). One may well feel that the orthodox medical views on the matter are brushed aside too lightly 'regardless of' the facts, which are said to have 'no bearing on the matter' and fail to 'carry weight', especially as the only medical evidence adduced to support their contentions is a single reference, and that to a letter written over three hundred years ago.

The unassailable fact regarding eating (and intravenous feeding) as opposed to intravenous transfusion of blood, is that these are entirely distinct physiological functions leading to different results. Intravenous feeding differs from oral feeding only in that the fluids introduced into the circulation are absorbed through the walls of the blood vessels instead of the alimentary tract. To summarise the two functions:

> Foodstuffs are metabolised by the body, and completely broken down in the process.
>
> Transfused blood is taken into the body unaltered and mixes with the recipient's own blood, continuing to function for a nearly normal lifespan. It is, in effect, a sort of tissue graft.

Consistent theology would require that if a prohibition exists on the eating of blood, then equally a similar prohibition must exist on the eating of fat, in the light of Leviticus 3: 16-17, '. . . all the fat is the Lord's. It shall be a perpetual statute for your generations throughout all your dwellings, that ye eat neither fat nor blood'. Yet this prohibition is one which is not mentioned in Jehovah's Witness literature: the reference is not even included in the otherwise very comprehensive list of 'Important Bible Words for Quick Reference' printed at the back of the Revised Version (1961) of the *New World Translation of the Holy Scriptures*. If there exists today a prohibition on blood and all blood components being taken into the body, then there must also exist a prohibition on all foodstuffs which include animal fats — butter, cream, milk, cheese, fat meat, lard, etc. and all items which include these. The fact that the Witnesses do not publicise such a prohibition again suggests that their reading of scripture is inconsistent. In conversation Jehovah's Witnesses usually agree that they 'try to avoid fat meat', but the question of other sources of fat, or of there being an absolute ban on eating it, is circumvented by the allegation that it was specifically the Mosaic Law (which included the ban on fat) which was abrogated by Christ's New Covenant, and that the ban on blood is a separate pre-Mosaic instruction given to Noah after the deluge, for all mankind. ('Only flesh with its soul, — its blood — YOU must not eat'. Gen. 9: 4 NW). Elsewhere Jehovah's Witnesses' literature states that: 'The condemning of murder and of use of blood as food God made a part of his covenant or solemn agreement with all mankind' (NHNE, p. 104). Yet the Witnesses agree that Christ, by His new covenant, abrogated the old covenant which no longer applies to Christians, nor even to the Jews (LGT, p. 183); they also state that: 'The law covenant cannot be taken apart, so that a part of it . . . could be abolished . . .' (LGT, p. 188). Christ summarised the whole law of His new covenant in a paraphrase on the Deuteronomic first commandment followed by the injunction, 'Thou shalt love thy neighbour as thyself. On these two commandments hang all the law and the prophets' (Mt. 22: 39-40). The clear implication is that the whole of the old law is abrogated, including the pre-Mosaic components.

Ever since the giving of the Mosaic Law the Jewish people have refrained from eating meat which has not been drained of blood, and also such products as blood-sausage which are made with whole blood, as of course they never accepted the Christian Gospel. That this law was always taken seriously is shown in the story related in Samuel. The people of Israel, after an exhausting battle against the Philistines, '. . . began darting greedily at the spoil and taking sheep and cattle and calves and slaughtering them on the earth, and the people fell to eating along with the blood' (1 Sam. 14: 32 NW). When this was brought to the notice of Saul he said '. . . Ye have transgressed . . .' (1 Sam. 14: 33) and promptly stopped the people, and made them kill the animals in front of him, draining the blood out properly.

It is in this ritual sense of eating only meat which has been drained of blood that Jehovah's Witnesses approach the application of this law to foodstuffs. 'If one learns that his butcher does not properly bleed the animals sold for food, he wisely finds another place to do business or even refains from eating those meats if nothing properly bled is available. Likewise, a conscientious person refrains from eating chicken or other meat in restaurants in places where he knows that little or no attention is given to the matter of proper bleeding. Under these circumstances, if a Christian wants to have meat in his diet he may buy a live animal or fowl and do the killing himself' (*Blood, Medicine and the Law of God,* p. 11). Now we remember that the law concerning blood is very strict. 'You must not eat any fat or any blood at all' (Lev. 3: 17 NW). Also the Jehovah's Witnesses take a very strict view about Bible interpretation: '. . . the Bible could not be all mixed up and allowing any interpretation to be made of it' (LGT, p. 8). In view of this we may reasonably expect that in following this law the Witnesses would avoid eating 'any blood at all'. It would not be sufficient that a formal and ritual draining of blood from a carcass be observed — if any blood at all should remain the meat may not, according to their own strict ruling, be eaten. Yet in the 'Questions from Readers' section in *Watchtower* the Witnesses are told, 'What God's law requires is that the blood be drained from the animal when it is killed, not . . . to draw out every trace of it'. 'It was not required that the meat be squeezed or that it be soaked; simply that the blood be poured out. If there is not enough blood to pour it out, Christians are not under obligation to take extreme measures to be sure that some blood is extracted' (*Watchtower,* Nov. 1, 1961, pp. 669-670). It would seem that once again we are faced with a situation where inconsistent theology can only be conformed to by a process of 'doublethink'.

The overall conclusion about Jehovah's Witness teaching on blood transfusion can only be that it is both inconsistent and unfounded.

Orthodox Christianity

The historical churches have never been faced with the problem of whether or not to accept blood transfusion, as there has never been any doubt that a measure which relieves suffering and saves life is right in the eyes of God. The whole concept of one man giving of his life blood to save another is bound up in three texts. 'For all the law is fulfilled in one word, even in this; Thou shalt love they neighbour as thyself' (Gal. 5: 14). 'Greater love hath no man than this, that a man lay down his life for his friends' (John 15: 13). '. . . God is love; and he that dwelleth in love dwelleth in God, and God in him' (1 John 4: 16).

If the scriptures fail to move a resolute Jehovah's Witness on this point one can only plead with him in the words of Cromwell. 'I beg you, by the bowels of Christ, consider you may be wrong'.

REFERENCES

All other references than those given below are given in full in the text.

THE BIBLE

Unless otherwise indicated all references are to the Authorised (Kings James) version.

Other translations are shown thus:

RV Revised Version

NEB New English Bible

NW New World Translation of the Holy Scriptures (Watchtower Bible and Tract Society) (Revised Edn., 1961).

JEHOVAH'S WITNESSES

LGT *Let God be True* (2nd Edn.) NHNE *New Heavens and a New Earth* *Blood, Medicine and the Law of God* *Watchtower* (periodical) *Awake!* (periodical)	Watch Tower Bible and Tract Society, New York and London

5

THE LEGAL POSITION

CONSIDERATION of the legal position in relation to refusal of blood transfusion falls into three sections:

(i) Action in respect of adults who refuse transfusion for themselves.

(ii) Action in respect of parents or guardians who refuse transfusions for children in their care.

(iii) Action against the parents or guardians of children who have died as a result of consent for transfusion being withheld.

In each case the legal position is not related solely to blood transfusion, but is part of the wider implications of medical treatment as a whole.

Action in respect of adults who refuse treatment for themselves. At first sight it would appear superfluous to consider whether or not an adult in full possession of his faculties has the legal right to accept or refuse any course of treatment advocated by his medical advisors. In the United Kingdom indeed there has, until recently, been no difficulty over this matter. If a doctor in general practice feels that a patient's refusal to accept the treatment advised leads to an untenable doctor-patient relationship he has, under the National Health Service Act, 1947, the right to have that patient's name removed from his list, subject to the moral obligation of ensuring, if the patient is at that time under treatment, that this may be continued under another practitioner. If the patient is unable to obtain acceptance on any other practitioner's list the local Executive Council may allocate him to a practitioner who is obliged to accept him. If a patient in hospital resolutely refuses a particular treatment then the next best alternative treatment — if any other exists — is offered. The general attitude in Britain is that expressed by Dr. Arthur Kelly of the Canadian Medical Association. 'Patient's have the right to accept or reject a doctor's advice according to their own desires. A doctor has no right to insist you accept his advice' (Toronto, Canada, *Globe and Mail*, April 15, 1960; *Canadian Doctor*, Dec. 1960, p. 49). The specific position in regard to blood transfusion in the United Kingdom has been very clearly expressed. 'In the event of a transfusion or other therapeutic measure of that type without consent, the aggrieved party would have the right to sue in the civil courts. Transfusion without consent is technically a "battery", a tort or civil wrong, and a trespass to the person. The first basic essential then of blood transfusion from the legal aspect is that it can only properly be carried out with real (explicit) consent (*Medicine, Science and the Law*, Jan., 1964).

The Medical Defence Union, in their booklet *Consent to Treatment*, give eminently sane and practical advice to doctors on the point.

'So far as adult patients are concerned (and in this context "adult" means over the age of sixteen) the physician or surgeon must realise that the adamant refusal of the patient to permit a blood transfusion under any circumstances place a restriction on him. It must remain for him to decide, in the exercise of his own professional conscience, whether or not he will treat the patient or operate under the limiting conditions propounded by the patient. If, and only if, the physician or surgeon decides to accept these limiting conditions, he should protect himself by adopting the procedure set out below. He should not agree to treat or operate on a patient who may require but will not accept a blood transfusion and who at the same time refuses to sign a conditional consent in the appropriate form referred to in paragraph (2) below. In this event he should make a full record of the facts in the clinical notes and this should be signed by him and by the witness who was present; he should also report the facts in writing to the hospital authority and make a full and immediate report to the patient's general practitioner.

The procedure referred to above is as follows:

1. the patient should be interviewed by the physician or surgeon in the presence of a witness. The patient should be given an unequivocal warning of the dangers that might arise as the result of his refusal to have a blood transfusion and an attempt should be made to persuade him to change his mind;

2. if the patient remained adamant he should be asked to sign a form acknowledging the fact that, although he has been warned that during the course of his treatment he may require a blood transfusion, he is unwilling to give his consent. The relevant form is form V or form VI, as the case may be, in the appendix to this memorandum.

FORM V. CONSENT TO OPERATIVE TREATMENT BY PATIENT WHO REFUSES TO HAVE A BLOOD TRANSFUSION

....Hospital.

I.................................. of.....................................
hereby give my consent to the performance upon me of the operation of ....,
the nature and effect of which have been explained to me by Dr/Mr .... and to the administration of a local or other anaesthetic. I also give my consent to the performance upon me of any other operative procedure which in the opinion of the surgeon it may be necesssary to perform upon me, without having obtained my express consent, during or by reason of the said operation or anything connected with it; except that, although it has been explained to me that in the course of or by reason of the said operation it may be necessary to give me a blood transfusion so as to render the operation successful, or to prevent injury to my health, or even to preserve my life, I hereby expressly withhold my consent to and forbid the administration to me of a blood transfusion in any circumstances or for any reason whatsoever and I accordingly absolve the surgeon, the hospital and every member of the medical staff concerned from all responsibility, and from any liability to me, or my estate, or to my dependants, or any damage or injury which may be caused to me, or to my estate, or to my dependents, in any way arising out of or connected with this my refusal to consent to any such blood transfusion.

Date........................ *(Signed)*..................................

Witnesses to patient's signature : ....

(Surgeon)

....

(Witness present at interview)

I confirm that I have explained to the patient the nature and effect of this operation and the possible risks attendant upon his refusal to accept a blood transfusion.

Date........................ *(Signed)*................................

FORM VI. CONSENT TO MEDICAL TREATMENT BY PATIENT WHO REFUSES TO HAVE A BLOOD TRANSFUSION

....Hospital

I.................................. of..................................

..................................acknowledge that I have been

informed that I am or may be suffering from ....

and that I require or may require treatment, the nature and

effect of which have been explained to me by Dr/Mr ....
I hereby give my consent to the administration of such medical treatment as the physician considers necessary; except that, although it has been explained to me that in the course of the said treatment it may be necessary to give me a blood transfusion so as to enhance the effectiveness of any treatment or even to preserve my life, I hereby expressly withhold my consent to and forbid the administration to me of a blood transfusion in any circumstances or for any reason whatsoever, and I accordingly absolve the physician, the hospital and every member of the medical staff concerned, from all responsibility, and from any liability to me, or to my estate, or to my dependants, or any damage or injury which may be caused to me, or to my estate or to my dependants, in any way arising out of or connected with this my refusal to consent to any such blood transfusion.

Date....................... *(Signed)*................................

Witness to patient's signature : ....
(Physician)

....
(Witness present at interview)

I confirm that I have explained to the patient the nature and effect of this treatment and the possible risks attendant upon his refusal to accept a blood transfusion.

Date....................... *(Signed)*................................

3. the patient's signature to the form should be witnessed by the physician or surgeon and the witness who was present at the interview.'

A recent British case has, however, raised some very important issues; notably the respect, or lack of it, given to a clear refusal to accept blood transfusion. The *Daily Mail* of November 6, 1970 carried the report that Mr. A. K., a nineteen-year-old Jehovah's Witness, had been admitted to Sheffield Royal Hospital three days previously with serious injuries sustained in a road accident. On arrival he refused blood transfusion and this attitude was later confirmed by his step-father and his mother. Eventually, during treatment, the patient was re-infused with two pints of his own blood (which had been collected during treatment) and then given another five units of blood. Despite treatment the patient died, and it was reported that the surgeon had told the parents 'he would go along with our wishes as far as he could but then he would have to give blood'. A Witness spokesman later commented, 'I am very surprised that the doctor took such a course. This has happened with children but not, as far as I know, with an adult. It really means that any adult who says he does not approve of a certain medical treatment can be overridden by a doctor. Doctors who do this are really putting themselves in the place of God'.

In the United States of America the position is not quite so clear, and there is evidence of conflicting legal opinions. As long ago as 1942 the Court of Appeals, District of Columbia, ruled in the case of *Bonner* vs *Moran:* 'We think there can be no doubt that a surgical operation is a technical battery, regardless of its results, and is excusable only when there is express or implied consent by the patient; or stated somewhat differently, the surgeon is liable in damages if the operation is unauthorized'. Generally speaking the American medical profession accept this principle, 'To administer to an individual or the junior members of his family a form of treatment which he has refused would constitute a violation of the patient's rights and could imply bodily assault' (*American Jnl. of Cardiology,* 1964, June). Recent events would suggest that these views are not universally held, and during the last few years there have been a crop of cases reported where medical authorities have sought court orders empowering them to carry out treatments against the patient's expressed wishes. In eight of the cases which the author has collected, consent was refused by the courts in only two. In one of the five cases where it was granted there are allegations of highly irregular procedures being employed in order to obtain consent, and in another the consent was subsequently ruled by a higher court to have been wrongly given. Because these cases are of such far-reaching and fundamental importance they are detailed below:

1. The first case, which appears to have established precedent in this matter, is particularly well documented having been taken on appeal as far as the U.S. Supreme Court. Mrs. J.L.J., aged 25, was admitted to Georgetown University Hospital with a bleeding ulcer. The patient, a Jehovah's Witness, refused to submit to blood transfusion and the hospital attorney requested a court order requiring the transfusion. An order was refused by District Judge Edward Tamm, but this

decision was overruled by Appeal Court Judge J. Skelly Wright who, after interviewing the patient, her husband and doctors, signed an order for the transfusion. In his memorandum on the decision Judge Wright said, 'I determined to act on the side of life. The Court was comforted by the apparent assurance from the patient herself, as well as from her husband, that if the Court undertook the responsibility for authorizing the transfusion, they themselves would not be in violation of their religious beliefs'. He also argued on two further aspects of the case. 'If it is unlawful for a parent to abandon a child, can a judge permit the ultimate abandonment of a child by the mother's voluntary death?' (N.B. In the United Kingdom the Suicide Act, 1961, sect. 1, enacted 'The rule of law whereby it is a crime to commit suicide is hereby abrogated'). After several transfusions, which replaced nearly two-thirds of her blood volume the patient recovered and after discharge from hospital asked for a hearing on the action, by the nine judges of the Circuit Court of Appeals of the District of Columbia, on a matter of personal principle. This court ruled that as the original order had by then expired, and Mrs. J. had left hospital, there was nothing to rehear. An appeal was then made to the United States Supreme Court, who refused to rule on the authority of Judge Wright to make the order. (Ref's. *Medical World News,* Nov. 8, 1963; *AMA News,* March 30, 1964; *Transfusion,* July/August, 1964: Sept./Oct., 1964).

2. A patient in Meadowbrook Hospital, Long Island, New York, refused a recommended treatment and the hospital authorities sought an order authorizing treat-

ment, from Judge B. S. Meyer of the Supreme Court. 'Judge Meyer remained unconvinced. The individual who is the subject of a medical decision, he declared, has the final say on that decision, " and must necessarily, in a system which gives the greatest possible protection to the individual in the furtherance of his own desire ".' (*Medical World News,* March 27, 1964). 'Pointing out that the patient was an adult in full possession of his faculties, Judge Meyer refused to issue the court order' (*Awake!* Sept. 8, 1964).

3. On May 16, 1964, at Anaheim, California, Mrs. R., a Jehovah's Witness, suffered a severe haemorrhage following childbirth, and refused transfusion. After several judges had refused to order a transfusion Judge H. S. Herlandes was contacted and gave an order *over the telephone.* There was no notice, no hearing, no witnesses called and no written order. An article in a Jehovah's Witness publication comments: 'Since when is a judge authorized to hold cases over the telephone? Since when is he authorized to make orders without all the evidence in front of him? The forms of legal procedure are a protection of fairness. Was this judge being fair? Was he even acting as a judge? If a judge puts his judicial gown on and goes out to participate in a lynching, is he still within the powers of his judicial office? Is a judicial assault done in defiance of the law and without any elementary pretense of the forms of law a judicial act?' (*Awake!* Sept. 8, 1964, p. 26). This summary raises some pertinent questions and would seem to be entirely reasonable.

4. At seven months of pregnancy obstetric complications indicated the probable necessity for Caesarian

section in Mrs. W.A., a Jehovah's Witness. Should such a procedure prove necessary, and should there be serious blood loss, the patient indicated that she was not prepared to receive a blood transfusion. The hospital attorney then applied to Judge L. Leonard of the New Jersey Supreme Court for authority to give a transfusion if necessary. Judge Leonard replied that he could find no power in the court 'that an adult person could be given medical treatment when he or she refused to accept the same'. On appeal to the New Jersey Supreme Court five days later, however, a ruling was given 'that since an unborn child was involved, a blood transfusion could be ordered. The Court provided for a guardian even though she had a competent husband. On June 25th her guardian (not her husband) ordered *one pint* of blood as she was delivered of her child by Caesarian section' (*Awake!* Sept. 8, 1964, p. 26). The decision of the New Jersey Court was subsequently upheld by the United States Supreme Court (*Transfusion,* Sept./Oct., 1964). This case has two particularly interesting features, *(i)* A court order was obtained on the grounds that a transfusion *might* become necessary in the future. There was no suggestion that it was at that time necessary to save life; *(ii)* In the event, a one-unit transfusion was given — a procedure which is widely deplored as generally being unnecessarily dangerous (see Chap. 3).

5. In New York a Jehovah's Witness patient with a bleeding ulcer was admitted to hospital. He consented to surgery but refused transfusion. The hospital applied to the Supreme Court judge in New York for authority to administer blood, but the judge pointed out that the

patient was an adult, fully capable of having the final say on his own decisions, and refused to sign an order. The patient died in the hospital about a week following surgery.

6. This case illustrates that court orders are not restricted to Jehovah's Witnesses refusing blood transfusion. Mrs. R.S., in hospital in Miami, Florida, was told that a gangrenous leg needed amputating. She refused consent and the hospital applied to Judge H. P. Dekle for an order authorizing the operation. The order was granted and the leg amputated (New York *Daily News,* July 20, 1964).

7. 'A court-ordered blood transfusion was judged an unconstitutional invasion of religious rights by the Illinois Supreme Court on March 18, 1965. The unanimous opinion of the court was that the lower court should not have permitted doctors to give the patient, Mrs. B.B., one of Jehovah's Witnesses, blood transfusions against her wishes. . . . Both Mrs. B. and her husband had signed waivers releasing the hospital from liability for her refusal to accept blood. Mrs. B. was being treated for a bleeding ulcer' (*Awake!* May 8, 1965). 'Coming to the heart of the matter, the decision said: "Applying the constitutional guarantees and the interpretation therefore heretofor enunciated to the facts before us, we find a competent adult who has steadfastly maintained her belief that acceptance of a blood transfusion is a violation of the law of God. Knowing full well the hazards involved, she has firmly opposed acceptance of such transfusions, notifying the doctor and the hospital of her convictions and desires,

and executing documents releasing both the doctor and the hospital from any civil liability which might be thought to result from a failure on the part of either to administer such transfusions. . . No overt act or affirmative act of appellants offers any clear and present danger to society — we have only a government agency compelling conduct offensive to appellant's religious principle. Even though we may consider appellant's beliefs unwise, foolish or ridiculous, in the absence of an overriding danger to society we may not permit interference therewith in the form of conservatorship established in the waning hours of her life for the sole purpose of compelling her to accept medical treatment forbidden by her religious principles, and previously refused by her with the full knowledge of the possible consequences. In the final analysis, what has happened here involves a judicial attempt to decide what course of action is best for a particular individual, not withstanding that individual's contrary views based upon religious convictions. Such action cannot be constitutionally countenanced." In conclusion the Supreme Court of Illinois stated that, "while the action of the circuit court herein was unquestionably well-meaning, . . . we have no recourse but to hold that it has interfered with basic constitutional rights"' (*Awake!* Aug. 8, 1965).

8. In Baltimore, Maryland, a 53-year-old woman was admitted to hospital and in view of her religious objections, and those of her husband, to receiving blood transfusions, a judge made a court order permitting the hospital to transfuse her. When the husband visited his wife in the hospital later he found her 'tied hand

and foot and being given blood transfusions' (*Awake!* 8 March 1968).

It would seem that the legal position in the United States is still not clear, in view of the conflicting decisions given by even the Supreme Court.

It is clearly the responsibility of those refusing blood transfusions to do so in a manner which admits of no doubt. This is normally done in writing, and the American Hospital Association recommended the use of a special form for this purpose based on the following example:

REFUSAL TO PERMIT BLOOD TRANSFUSION

I request that no blood or blood derivatives be administered

to ....

during this hospitalization. I hereby release the hospital, its personnel, and the attending physician from any responsibility whatever for unfavourable reactions or any untoward results due to my refusal to permit the use of blood or its derivatives and I fully understand the possible consequences of such refusal on my part.

It is suggested that the form show the name of hospital and the date, and be signed by the patient, and his/her spouse if married. In the case of a minor the signature of a parent or guardian, witnessed, and with an indication of relationship or status, would be acceptable. In order to indicate their wishes in case of emergency, Jehovah's Witnesses carry a card on their person stating 'No Blood Transfusion'.

Arising out of one of the American cases cited (No. 1) an interesting point in British law may be worth consideration. In his decision Judge Wright said, 'If suicide is illegal, can a judge allow a hospital patient to choose death by refusing medical treatment? '. As has been pointed out, under British law, section 1 of the Suicide Act, 1961, made suicide no longer a crime. However, section 2 of the Act states, 'A person who aids, abets, counsels or procures the suicide of another, or an attempt by another to commit suicide shall be liable on conviction on indictment to imprisonment for a term not exceeding fourteen years'. Suicide may be committed by acts of commission or omission (e.g. refusing to eat) and it could be argued that by refusing to accept a blood transfusion when *in extremis,* and in full knowledge of the probable consequences of the results of such refusal, one would be in fact committing suicide. In such a circumstance would the doctor accepting such a refusal be guilty of aiding and abetting the suicide?; and would the Watchtower Bible and Tract Society, who teach the precepts leading to such a refusal, be guilty of counselling the suicide? Such questions have never so far arisen in the British courts. It is to be hoped that they never do.

Action in respect of parents or guardians who refuse transfusion for children in their care. The position in respect of minors requiring blood transfusion is rather different from that with adults. A child for all practical purposes is any person from the moment of birth up to the age of 16. The Family Law Reform Act, 1969, fixed the legal age of majority in England and Wales as 18, but also provided for consent to medical treatment to be given at 16. Up to these ages consent required for any purpose is to be given by the parent or legal guardian. Legal provision to ensure the welfare of children was originally incorporated in the Poor Law Amendment Act, 1868, under which it was an offence for any person 'wilfully to neglect to provide adequate food, clothes, medical aid or lodging' for his child, whereby the child 'should be, or should be likely to be, seriously injured'. This section was repealed and replaced by the Prevention of Cruelty to Children Act, 1894, under which any person having the custody or care of a child was guilty of a misdemeanour if he or she 'wilfully neglects such child in a manner likely to cause such child unnecessary suffering or injury to its health'. Although there was no specific reference to medical aid in this latter Act its intention was clearly defined in 1899 in the Court of Crown Cases Reserved by Lord Russell of Killowen, L.C.J., who pointed out that 'it would be an odd result if we were obliged to come to the conclusion that in dealing with such a subject as the protection of children the law had meant to take what may be described as a retrograde step'. (*R* v *Senior,* 1899, IQB, 283). The present position is covered by sect. 1 of the Children and Young Persons Act, 1933, which makes it a criminal offence 'if any person over the age of sixteen who has the custody, charge, or care of any child under that age, wilfully assaults, ill-treats, neglects, abandons, or exposes him . . . in a manner likely to cause him unnecessary suffering or injury to health'. In the case of *Regina v Senior* referred to above it was laid down by Mr. Justice Wills and Lord Russell that by 'wilful' it was necessary to understand that the act was committed deliberately and intentionally, not by accident or inadvertance, but in a fully conscious manner. By negligence it was necessary to understand the refusal to give reasonable care, that is to say, the omission of the measures which every reasonable parent would give in the ordinary course of human life.

The position on age of consent in England and Wales was stated in the Family Law Reform Act, 1969, which reduced the age of majority from 21 to 18. Section 8 of that Act also effectively reduced further the age at which consent may be given to medical treatment. It was stated that: 'The consent of a minor who has attained the age of sixteen years to any surgical, medical or dental treatment which, in the absence of consent, would constitute a trespass to his person, shall be as effective as it would be if he were of full age; and where a minor has by virtue of this section given an effective consent to any treatment it shall not be necessary to obtain any consent for it from his parent or guardian'. The Act did not, however, make any explicit provision for the age at which any particular medical treatment may be *refused;* thus acceptance by a 16 year old of a transfusion, despite parental objections, would appear to be valid, although the converse situation of a refusal of treatment where the parent, guardian, or local authority (or court) in whose care the 16 year old may have been put, wish the treatment, is more obscure.

In recent years the refusal of a parent or guardian to allow an operation upon a child has come before the courts. In such cases courts must 'consider the nature of the operation and the reasonableness of the refusal' (*Oakley v Jackson* (1914) 1. KB. 216). In 1912, magistrates convicted a father of neglecting to provide medical aid when he refused to allow his child to be operated upon for cleft palate. Offences involving cruelty to children are both indictable and summary.

The maximum punishment is two years imprisonment, a fine of £100, or both. Upon summary conviction the maximum is six months imprisonment, a fine of £25, or both (*The Criminal Law* by F. T. Giles, 1952, Penguin, Middlesex).

Quite clearly there is a legal obligation on parents to permit such medical treatment to their children as may be reasonably felt necessary for relief of pain or to save life. In any case where a parent refuses to permit such a measure it is open to the courts to transfer the child to the care of the local authority, or to make him a ward of the court. The fact that an older child may concur in the parents' refusal of a particular treatment has no bearing on the case, as is illustrated by a recent case in Norwich. A 14-year-old girl, a Jehovah's Witness, whose parents were both also of that faith, was admitted to West Norwich Hospital in a critical condition following an internal haemorrhage due to a perforated gastric ulcer. It was feared by the doctors that a further haemorrhage might prove fatal, and decided that a transfusion was essential. As the parents refused consent a special meeting of Norwich Juvenile Court was called to hear an application by the hospital secretary. Evidence was taken in the Court-room and at the bedside of the patient who herself, despite her weak state, indicated that she did not want a transfusion. The magistrates then made an order placing the girl in the care of Norfolk County Council and the Council's deputy Children's Officer immediately agreed to a transfusion which was given, the child subsequently recovering. At a Juvenile Court hearing eight weeks later, when the order was revoked, the girl said, 'I would rather have died than gone against my faith. I want the whole world to know that I did not want that transfusion and would not have it again' (*Scottish Daily Mail,* Sept. 19 and Nov. 10, 1964). In the case of newborn children, such as those requiring exchange transfusion for haemolytic disease of the newborn, similar procedures apply. In emergencies there may not be time to convene a special court and in such cases doctors are advised to obtain a second medical opinion and, that if transfusion were then agreed upon, official action for assault would not be taken. In such circumstances there would of course be nothing to prevent the parents applying to a magistrate for a summons against the doctor performing the transfusion, or even removing the child from the hospital. In the latter case they may be laying themselves open to a charge of wilful neglect.

A somewhat different problem may arise in circumstances in which an adult is temporarily standing *in loco parentis* to a child who is a Jehovah's Witness (as may happen with the Principal of a boarding school, for example). Should such a child require urgent medical treatment involving administration of a blood transfusion the adult who is *in loco parentis* has a duty to see that the child receives all necessary medical attention advised by the doctor in charge of the case. If, however, the parent has expressly and unequivocally stated in writing that the child is, under no circumstances whatever, to receive a blood transfusion, then the adult in charge of the child should advise the medical staff concerned, making it clear that he is not personally refusing consent, but that he has no authority from the parents to give it. It will then be up to the doctor concerned to decide whether or not to ignore the parental refusal to consent, or to apply for a court order placing the child in the custody of the court, who may order the transfusion to proceed if it thinks fit. This latter course of action, as is made clear elsewhere, the author does not believe to be satisfactory. The moral dilemma in this case is that the doctor or hospital official, while believing the parental attitude to be wrong, has no opportunity to reason with the parents in an attempt to change their opinion.

The converse situation — a Jehovah's Witness in the position of Principal of a school, or for other reasons *in loco parentis* to children who are not Witnesses — may also pose problems in emergency situations where consent to blood transfusion as treatment is required. As was pointed out in Chapter 4, Jehovah's Witnesses are employed as nurses, doctors, pathologists, etc., and in these capacities are inevitably required to be involved in blood transfusion administered to non-Witness patients. By the same arguments used ('. . . the Christian is not responsible for the worldly misuse of blood'. *Watchtower,* Nov. 15, 1964) it is to hoped that a Witness *in loco parentis* to a non-Witness child requiring transfusion would not specifically forbid a transfusion for that child in emergency. If this were done the doctor concerned would again have to consider whether he should over-ride the instruction in the interests of the child. Should a child suffer or die as a result of consent for a transfusion being withheld by a Jehovah's Witness who has temporary custody of that child, then the Witness would be open to prosecution on a criminal charge as well as any civil action for damages brought by the parent.

In answer to a question in the House of Commons, former Minister of Health, Mr. Kenneth Robinson, has stated the Ministry's views. He said that hospital authorities have been advised not to resort to the courts, but to rely on the clinical judgements of the consultants concerned after full discussion with the parents. He further said that he was advised that if a transfusion was given against the wishes of parents, providing that the practitioner concerned had obtained the written supporting opinion of a colleague that the patient's life was in danger, and an acknowledgement from the parents that they refused consent, despite their having been given an explanation of the danger, there would be little risk in a court of law if the doctor had acted with due professional competence and in accordance with his own professional conscience. It must be pointed out, however, that this is the opinion of a Minister given to Parliament, and may or may not be supported by a court of law. (Parliamentary Debates: *Hansard,* House of Commons Official Report, Vol. 724, No. 47, Monday, 14 February 1966.)

The attitude of the Medical Defence Union towards transfusion of children with Jehovah's Witness parents is again a model of sanity and reason. Their advice to doctors is: 'It is generally believed that the administration of a blood transfusion to a child in opposition to the parents' wishes constitutes an assault in law. It may be that common law will protect a doctor who acts competently and in good faith in such a situation. Despite the fact that the administration of a blood transfusion to a child in opposition to the parents' wishes may constitute a technical assault, it is unlikely that any injury or damage to the child could be proved. The worst that could happen in such a case would be an action for assault but, where the alternative to a blood transfusion is death or serious impairment of health, it is highly improbable that any such action would succeed. In such cases the Council of the Medical Defence Union is of the opinion that the practitioner should follow the dictates of his professional conscience. Any member of the Union may rest assured that if he finds himself in difficulty arising out of his decision to give a blood transfusion to a child, despite the expressed opposition of the parents, he may count on the full support of the Union.

In some cases a procedure has been used which involves the removal of the child from the custody of its parents under the Children and Young Persons Acts. The Union does not favour this procedure for children in hospital'.

In the United States similar provisions regarding minors apply although not so many cases can be traced in the literature. In a case in Illinois in 1953, a newborn infant was made a ward of the court in order that a transfusion could be administered, and in 1960 an unusual case occurred in Indiana when Judge R. Groover issued a restraining order to prevent two parents, who were Witnesses, from interfering with medical aid for their then unborn child, who was expected to be affected with haemolytic disease of the newborn. (*AMA News,* Feb. 8, 1960). In Cleveland, Ohio, in 1963, a court order was granted to permit an operation in the case of a 14-year-old girl with cancer of the hip, the mother having refused consent (Toronto *Globe and Mail,* Nov. 12, 1963).

One relevant point made by Jehovah's Witnesses, in the context of the commercial health service in the U.S.A. is worth noting in passing. 'When a court removes the child from the custody of its parents and appoints a guardian for the child for the purpose of giving a child a blood transfusion, the guardian has the child treated according to his wishes. Then the hospital and the doctors are no longer acting as employees of the parent but of the guardian. Should not the guardian then be required to pay all the hospital, doctor and blood transfusion bills? He is the one that ordered the treatment is he not? And in the event the child dies, should not the one acting as guardian be required to take care of the funeral expenses? ' (*Awake!* March 8, 1968). It seems a valid point.

In Canada a number of cases have occurred of children being given court-ordered blood transfusions. One particular case occasioned world-wide press coverage due to the indecorous manner in which hospital staff attempted to impose their wishes. A baby born at Smiths Falls hospital, in Ontario, on April 1, 1970, was believed to require an exchange transfusion on her second day after birth. The mother had already indicated that she would not consent to transfusion and, during her temporary absence from the hospital (to attend a court hearing, concerning divorce from her husband) the child was removed by the Childrens' Aid Society to the Kingston General Hospital some sixty miles away. The mother drove to that hospital accompanied by her parents and brothers and was told by a doctor, ' I am going to give that child a blood transfusion if I have to go to jail for it '. The mother decided to go elsewhere for treatment but the doctor and two other members of the hospital staff attempted to physically prevent the mother and child leaving. The mother got her baby out into a waiting car but the doctor struggled with one of the men in the party, right out onto the pavement outside the building.

A warrant was issued to search the mother's home and then the Crown Attorney ordered it to be cancelled. The Children's Aid Society applied for a court order to make them guardians but the judge refused to act until 'proper procedures were put before him'. The Crown Attorney, while commending the action of the doctor who had delivered the baby, went on to admit 'the mother had an equal right to remove the child from the hospital'. A great deal of press activity followed (largely instigated by the doctor who had wished to administer the transfusion) but the child survived without treatment and subsequently appeared with her mother and a legal counsel, on television to explain what had happened, despite the doctor's comment previously that 'there is a good chance it is dead'. In this case the refusal of the courts to be stampeded resulted in a happy outcome, although the dignity of the medical profession was hardly enhanced.

In Australia parents' consent for transfusion of a child is no longer required.

The whole position of Jehovah's Witnesses being forced by American courts to accept transfusion was brought to a head in 1965 by a petition filed in the federal court to prevent doctors, hospitals and judges from making Witnesses submit to blood transfusions. The petition cited seventeen cases during the preceding six years of transfusions being forced on members, especially children, and contended that this practice violated the constitutional right of their members to religious liberty. The suit also criticized the practice of judges in declaring children wards of court so that transfusions can be given against the parents' wishes, and asked that the federal court find that ' members of the group have a right to raise their children in the " teachings, discipline and practices " of their religion and to care for their families according to their " own best judgment of the family welfare ",' (*Spokane Daily Chronicle,* Nov. 18, 1965, reported in ' Transfusion ', Vol. 6, p. 81, 1966). The case was finally argued before a three-judge United States District Court in Seattle, Washington, between 19-21 June 1967. Directed particularly to the practice in Washington state, whereby removal of children from Jehovah's Witness parents by the courts, in cases where blood transfusions may be indicated, had become ' almost standard procedure ' (*Awake!* September 22, 1967), the action was against twenty-two individual physicians, ten hospitals, sixteen executives, six judges, the attorney general, a probation officers and two lawyers who had been directly involved in recent cases. The complaint also sought a permanent injunction against the entire medical profession and judicial system in Washington state to restrain them from forcing blood transfusions upon Jehovah's Witnesses ' in violation of their Constitutional rights '. The judges hearing the case were Judge Lindberg (presiding) and Judges Hambly and Becks. A number of witnesses were called for both sides and in their final arguments the attorneys for the plaintiffs stressed that they were not seeking financial damages, but relief from a practice which they held to be unconstitutional. After five months of deliberation, on November 20, a decision was handed down which rejected the petition. Among other things ' The three judges . . . ruled yesterday that no rights under the Constitution are abridged by the state law' (*Seattle Times,* November 21, 1967). It was judged that: 'The overwhelming weight of medical opinion is that blood transfusions are necessary in certain cases to save lives, and, in fact, do save lives'. The court did not comment on whether refusing consent to transfusion of a minor constitutes gross and wilful neglect, for which purpose the statute in question had been enacted.

Jehovah's Witnesses appealed against the District Court judgement but on April 8, 1968, the United States Supreme Court, by a 7 to 2 majority, refused to hear the case and on May 27 denied a petition for it to be re-heard. It would appear from this case that in the United States the law is not prepared to hear protests on matters of religious conscience, when these are contrary to general and 'non-sectarian' medical opinion. An article in *Awake!* (July 8, 1968) reminded its readers that for a considerable time 'non-sectarian medical opinion' authorized the use of thalidomide during pregnancy — and of the consequences of that opinion. The court was seemingly uninfluenced by either medical or religious views submitted by the plaintiffs and found that courts were right in enforcing this particular treatment against the wishes of patients, or their parents. The confirmation of this finding by the Supreme Court appears to finalise the matter.

It is interesting to note that the Newark, New Jersey *Star Ledger* of November 26, 1967 (i.e. six days after the District Court's decision, referred to above, reported that 'a small businessman and his wife stood by while their five-year-old adopted daughter succumbed to bronchial pneumonia.' They did not summon medical aid because they were Christian Scientists. The court found no reason to act, although the Essex County prosecutor had asked for an opinion 'on the basis of a recent case of Jehovah's Witnesses where the court did act'.

Action against the parents or guardians of children who have died as a result of consent for transfusion being withheld. In the United Kingdom, apart from the possibility of action brought under the Children and Young Persons Act, 1933, a parent who permits the death of a child due to withholding medical aid may be charged with manslaughter. Manslaughter is the killing of another person unlawfully, and may be voluntary or involuntary. 'Involuntary manslaughter occurs where one person is killed because someone else has acted in an unlawful manner, but without intending to kill or hurt anyone' (*The Criminal Law* by F. T. Giles, 1954, Penguin, Middlesex). The offence is triable only by Crown Courts and the maximum penalty is life imprisonment.

The precedent-setting case is *Regina v Senior* (1899), IQB, 283. Mr. Senior belonged to the Peculiar People, a religious body now known as the Union of Evangelical Churches. One of the tenets of this church was in the efficacy of prayer and laying-on of hands to effect healing, and consequently the members refused to accept orthodox medical aid. Mr. Senior's son died of diarrhoea, for which he had received no medical treatment, and Senior was convicted of manslaughter by reason of 'wilful neglect', as understood in Sect. 1 of the Prevention of Cruelty to Children Act, 1894. In view of the importance of the case on grounds of principle, Senior having pleaded that medical treatment was contrary to his religious principles, the case went to the High Court where the conviction was upheld. Mr. Justice Wills and Lord Russell of Killowen held that whatever his motives Senior was guilty of wilful negligence.

A similar position exists in Canada where precedent was set in the case of *R. v. Lewis.* Under the Criminal Code of Canada (Statutes of Canada, 55 & 56 Vict., c. 29, s. 210, sub-s. [1]). Lewis, a Christian Scientist, had been convicted of manslaughter following his failure to provide medical aid for his child. The Hon. Charles Moss, Chief Justice of the Court of Appeal, Ontario, commented on the provisions of the statute which required that: 'Everyone who is a parent, guardian, or head of a family, is under a legal duty to provide necessaries for any child under the age of sixteen years, is criminally responsible for omitting, without lawful excuse, to do so while such child remains a member of his or her household, whether such child is helpless or not, if the death of such child is caused or if his life is endangered or his health is or is likely to be permanently injured by such omission'. It was agreed that 'necessaries' included medical treatment, and at the same time confirmed that the motives or good faith of the prisoner were not material to the case. The conviction was upheld.

In Australia, Alvin Jehu, a migrant from England and a Jehovah's Witness, was convicted of manslaughter in Melbourne in 1959 following the death of his child due to refusal to consent to a blood transfusion. As a result Australian law was changed so that in emergencies parental consent for blood transfusion of a child is no longer necessary.

6

THE ETHICAL AND MORAL ARGUMENTS

HAVING read the preceding chapters one may perhaps wonder what is the problem? On medical grounds blood transfusion can generally be justified; the theological objections to the use of blood can be met and countered; the law is clear on the duties of a parent to its child. Yet it is at this point that the most difficult aspects of this study arise.

If, taking all factors into account, one feels that it is essential that a child, for example, should be transfused but the parent refuses consent, is it morally right that the force of law should be invoked to compel submission to that treatment? In actual practice it usually is a child who is involved in cases where resort is had to law, and in such cases it is usually difficult to separate ethical judgment from pure emotion. The majority of people of all types — doctors, nurses, priests, and laymen and women — with whom the author has discussed this matter have started by saying that of course recourse should be had to law to permit transfusion of a child if the parents refuse. When some of the ethical problems involved have been pointed out to them, most have become less certain. Many have ended by adopting the opposite stand that such compulsion can not be justified, thus indicating that the ethical problems are not widely enough appreciated.

Essentially the problem presents itself in two halves; cases involving adults, and those involving children. As will be shown, however, certain basic common principles are involved.

In the case of adults it is difficult to argue with the premise that any adult in full possession of his faculties has the right to accept or reject any particular form of medical treatment offered to him. This right is widely recognised already in the case of Roman Catholics, whose faith forbids them to practise or accept therapeutic abortion, artificial insemination (with one minor exception), artificial methods of birth control, caesarian section (except when vaginal delivery would constitute a serious hazard to the life of the woman or the child), craniotomy and embryotomy in obstetric practice, electro-convulsive therapy, euthanasia, leucotomy and sterilization. By the same token it is difficult to understand why a Jehovah's Witness should not be allowed similar freedom to refuse blood transfusion. The reason for the refusal is immaterial. In the United States it appears that some authorities feel otherwise and, as the examples given in Chapter 5 illustrate, the force of law has been invoked to compel submission to blood transfusion and to amputation. Further to this point one must consider the 'moral blackmail' which may be applied. While it is right that a doctor should do all in his power to try to persuade a patient to accept a treatment which he, the doctor, feels to be necessary, is it right for him to refuse all further treatment to that patient if permission is still withheld? It would seem not, but this is not infrequently the case in the United

States (*Blood, Medicine and the Law of God*, pp. 47-51). In Britain, the ethically acceptable solution has generally been applied of providing the next best treatment, if any. Acceptance of a patient's wishes in matters of religious conscience should take into account the necessity of regarding the total welfare of the patient, which includes his spiritual welfare and integrity (*Surgery, Gynaecology and Obstetrics*, Apr. 1959)

The recent British case involving over-riding of an adult's wishes (referred to in Chapter 5) raises again the ethical situation of doctors who disregard the Medical Defence Union's advice to accept the patient's restriction on treatment or to hand over the case to another practitioner who will do so. One hopes that the case will prove to have been an isolated one. Of almost unbelievable arrogance in this case was the remark of a senior hospital administrator that 'there are occasions when a surgeon has to act like this. We are more concerned with a boy's life than with a father's conscience'. The Family Law Reform Act of 1970 set the age of majority in Britain at eighteen. A man of nineteen has an undeniable right in the free democracy of this country to accept or reject any medical treatment offered to him, and it may be commented that any thinking person concerned with personal freedom is more concerned with a man's rights, than with a hospital administrator's (or doctor's) conscience.

The attitude sometimes adopted in the United States is illustrated by a case reported in Jehovah's Witness literature in recent years. In December 1964 Mrs. S.C., a former nurse, was admitted to the St. Frances Cabrini Hospital for a hysterectomy (removal of the uterus). She signed a document releasing the surgeon and the hospital from any liability resulting from a failure to administer blood, and the surgeon agreed to perform the operation without the use of blood. When Mrs. S.C. awoke from the anaesthetic she found that a blood transfusion was being administered and the surgeon explained to her that 'this is often done to Jehovah's Witnesses without their knowledge' (*Awake!* September 22, 1967).

In considering whether or not the force of law should be applied to an adult refusing treatment, there are arguments in favour of so doing. The individual is a member of the community. This is a two-way relationship, the individual needing the community, which provides him with the necesities of life and with a (relatively) safe and stable environment in which to live his life; conversely the community is no more than the sum total of a number of individuals and needs the individual for survival. The community cannot afford to allow itself to disintegrate and so cannot afford to allow individual members the right of self destruction. We shall return to this point later.

One further aspect of this problem is also worth considering. In his judgement on case 1, cited in the previous chapter, Judge Wright said: 'If it is unlawful for a parent to abandon a child, can a judge permit the ultimate abandonment of a child by the mother's voluntary death?' (*Transfusion,* 1964, 4, p. 187). Leaving aside the question of whether it is lawful, one may well question whether this would constitute a morally justifiable act. Particularly if the individual should be the only surviving parent of that child. To abandon a child by allowing one's own death would surely be an act of mental cruelty to the child that would constitute a far greater crime against the conscience than would a breach of a religious law. It would indeed be an act of gross selfishness in placing the parent's own soul before the child's. Such consideration may well be put, and indeed should be put, to the patient, but they are scarcely grounds for making the parent's decision for him by process of law.

When considering the question of children the position is more complicated. Amongst the Jews, and subsequently among the Christian church which grew out of Judaism, great stress has always been laid upon the family as the important unit of society. In the ten commandments children were adjured to 'Honour thy father and thy mother . . .' (Ex. 20: 12), and in the proverbs of Solomon we read the injunction to parents to 'Train up a child in the way he should go . . .' (Prov. 22: 6), because 'A wise son maketh a glad father: but a foolish son is the heaviness of his mother' (Prov. 10: 1). This reciprocal duty between parents and children is at the basis of our society today, whether we be Jew, Christian or atheist. Parents have the moral responsibility to care for their children and to do that which they believe to be right and best for the child. This freedom of the parent to choose what is best for his child is demonstrated in Britain in the case of vaccination and immunisation. Medical science has proved that these procedures are of prime importance to the community in keeping the incidence of such deadly diseases as diphtheria, poliomyelitis, etc., at a low level, and the vast majority of parents agree with the need and arrange for their children to be immunised. The State recognises the right of freedom of choice for the individual in these matters however, and any parent who for any reason does not wish his child to be protected has the right to refuse consent. The community may deplore such a refusal, but it nevertheless permits it as part of the price paid by the society in a free country for individual freedom of choice, even though the child is more likely to suffer if it subsequently contracts the disease, and may die of it. By an extension of this principle one must grant, especially in a country where religious freedom and tolerance is one of the great liberties allowed to the individual, that a parent has the right — even the duty — to make all the decisions for his child regarding medical treatment; particularly is this so if the treatment in question is so contrary to the individual's beliefs as to represent in his eyes a peril to the soul. Whether or not the belief is acceptable to the majority is immaterial, if it is firmly and honestly held by the individual in question. The rest of society may be right — but they may be wrong. It is here that individual freedom of choice becomes so important a liberty.

Here again arguments may be made for the opposite viewpoint. As with the adult, so is each child a member of the community, and the community has the duty to conserve the lives of its members. It is at this point that we reach one of the most critical questions. What is the community? Is it the State, or is it the family unit? To which of these levels of community does the individual's greatest loyalty lie? Which type of community is the more important? If we claim that the State is the more important unit of society, then obviously this means that the welfare of the individual — whether it be his physical or his spiritual welfare — is the concern of the State, which must be prepared to overrule the parent if his views on what constitutes the welfare of his child do not conform with the views of the State (that is, with the majority of its members). If on the other hand the family is the more important unit then clearly responsibility for the welfare of a child lies solely with its parents. Unfortunately it is not quite as simple as this, as each State has members who are demonstrably incapable of exercising their responsibilities to their family; it is for this reason that laws have been found necessary to prevent cruelty to children by their parents, and to ensure that parents provide all the 'necessaries' for their children.

Let us then agree that it is the responsibility of parents to provide for their children's physical welfare, and the responsibility of the State to ensure that this is adequately done. What then of a child's spiritual welfare? In a State where religious freedom and tolerance are important parts of the constitution, this can only be the duty of the parents. (The State may indeed provide a guide, in the form of Bible study classes in its schools as is done in Britain, but it cannot compel attendance at these lessons.) But what is the position when something which the State considers necessary for the physical welfare of a child is considered by the parents to be contrary to that child's spiritual welfare? This is exactly the position in regard to blood transfusion with Jehovah's Witnesses. No matter what the medical indication for a transfusion may be, Jehovah's Witnesses firmly and honestly believe that God said '. . . I shall certainly set my face against the soul that is eating the blood, and I shall indeed cut him off from amongst his people' (Lev. 17: 10 NW). To these people a blood transfusion imperils the soul and its prospects of everlasting life. This is something that Jehovah's Witnesses who are loving parents will not risk for their child, even if the consequence is a shortening of the child's earthly life. It cannot be claimed that a Witness who refuses a transfusion for his child is lacking in loving care for the child. Indeed such a heartrending decision can only be made out of deep love for the child, and for what the parent believes to be the will of God. The individual, be he doctor, hospital official, children's officer, magistrate or judge, who presumes to over-rule a man's conscience on such a vital matter is setting himself on a level with God. St. Paul said 'Let us not therefore judge one another any more: but judge this rather, that no man put a stumbling block or an occasion to fall in his brother's way' (Rom. 14: 13). In the sermon on the mount Jesus said 'Judge not, that ye be not judged' (Matt. 7: 1). In matters of the spirit there can be no better advice.

How then are we to regard the situation where one parent holds religious views which will not permit transfusion, while the other does not? The position where a Jehovah's Witness is married to someone who is not of this faith. It is tempting to take the easy way out by saying that consent could be given by the one parent, thus removing the necessity for recourse to the law. While this is true it does nothing to suggest a solution for the parents themselves, who face an *impasse* where both love their child and wish to do the best thing for it, but their ideas of what constitutes the best thing are diametrically opposed. In such a case the ethical problem facing the community at large is indeed solved if one parent consents, as the community that is the State is not thrown into conflict with the community of the family. Within the family, however, the conflict is probably worsened by such an action. If one doubts the mental turmoil which is engendered in such a situation the author would suggest that they read the novel '*Life for Ruth*', and if possible see the film of the same name upon which William Drummond based it. In this story just such a situation arises and, while the situation between the parents is resolved by a rather artificial literary twist, the problems are most realistically illustrated. (This book also illustrates the tragic complications that ensue for all concerned when the problem is viewed purely as an emotional one.) The differences between the parents in such a case are essentially religious ones and can only be solved by religion, and with a knowledge of the faith of one another, and of the reasons for it. Local ministers may not prove of too much assistance in this latter context as each is likely to be too deeply committed to their own viewpoint to be able to appreciate or have any sympathy with the other. Also one must sadly admit that each is likely to be in too great a degree of ignorance of the basic tenets and beliefs of the other's faith to act successfully as intermediary in such an inter-family problem. It is possible that this book may help to disperse some of these fogs of doubt. In any case one can offer no better advice to those involved in such a tragic situation than to try the power of prayer. The ethical problem of whether the parent who does not object to blood transfusion should give his consent, in the face of his spouse's opposition, is not simple. It can only be taken in the light of the faith of the individual. If there is such a thing as a 'right' course it is probably to act, in the words of Judge Skelly Wright, 'on the side of life'.

If as Christians we believe that God is Love, then we cannot believe that a child's soul would suffer for our act: if we do not believe in God, then we can give consent with a clear personal conscience.

On the purely religious aspect of this problem there is indeed consolation to be offered to the parent who is over-ruled by the law of the State or by his husband or wife. Jesus said '. . . it is impossible but that offences will come: but woe unto him, through whom they come!' (Luke 17: 1). He also said '. . . Render to Caesar the things that are Caesar's, and to God the things that are God's . . .' (Mk. 12: 17). If the Jehovah's Witness believes that a blood transfusion given against His will is rendering to Caesar the things that are God's, then the fault before God will be that of the one causing the transfusion rather than the one receiving it. This attitude is, in practice, taken by Jehovah's Witnesses. The Christian magistrate making an order under these circumstances would also do well to remember the effects on his own soul if in fact an offence is being committed before God. The other parent giving consent will have already considered this.

There is a further aspect of compulsion in applying medical aid that merits serious consideration, and this applies whether the patient is a child or an adult. It is simply the freedom of the individual. Once one allows the principle that an individual has the right to choose for himself, then any action which over-rules that right is liable to become the thin end of a long wedge. We have already seen how this is working in practice in the United States (see Chapter 5). The over-ruling of a parent's decision in regard to its child is extended to over-ruling the adult's decision in regard to himself. The over-ruling in respect of a minority religious belief is extended to over-ruling the whole principle of an adult being allowed to accept or reject a particular form of medical treatment (see case 6 cited in Chapter 5). The State is gradually taking over the function of making decisions for the individual. It is in this way that free countries cease to be free and become totalitarian. It was indeed by the taking-over of the German children into the Hitler Youth movement that freedom and privacy were finally suppressed in Nazi Germany. This is not mere fanciful speculation. Freedom is a precious and comparatively rare possession, to be jealously guarded in those countries where it exists. Any one encroachment on individual liberty is one too many, and where the security and peace of the state is not involved, cannot be justified.

The Montana Law Review, Vol. 26 (1964), pp. 103-104, discusses cases involving blood transfusion and Jehovah's Witnesses, and in case No. 4 listed in Chapter 5 concludes that the Court's decision ' is too dangerous to be allowed as precedent '. It further points out that to condone such legislation ' it would have to be argued that in certain situations a particular religious belief makes a person " Incompetent " and powerless to help himself, and that the state, as *parens patriae*, may assume temporary jurisdiction for the person's own benefit. This would open the door to further expansion of the state's power to regulate individuals, and worse, to regulate religious belief. If the state could hold a religious belief as making a person incompetent, could not the state then actually circumvent the constitutional ban on interfering with the belief itself? The concept of the state stepping into a person's religious life " for his own good" is repugnant to the spirit of the first amendment. As the law stands today, there is no legal justification for this kind of interference, and the expansion of any of the doctrines discussed, in any general way, would be an excessive infringement upon the personal liberties of the individual guaranteed under the first amendment'.

The position has been admirably summarised by Father John C. Ford, S.J., in an article in the *Linnacre Quarterly,* which was subsequently reprinted by the American Association of Blood Banks. 'State power is exaggerated when one subscribes to the proposition that any interference by the State can be justified as long as the majority approves. Democracy does not mean that the majority is right, but majority rule is a practical way of making a republic work. If it were true that mere force of numbers made the difference between right and wrong, good and bad, then mere force would be controlling. Might would make right. But if anything is clear in the fundamental political thought of our country, it is the idea that minorities have a right to exist and to propagate their ideas. It was a minority that thought slavery wrong and finally abolished it. Right and wrong are not determined by a show of hands but by a show of minds' (Bulletin AABB, 9, p. 27, 1956).

In considering these matters one is bound to recall the whole principle of democracy as compressed into the immortal phrase of Voltaire. 'I disapprove of what you say, but I will defend to the death your right to say it.'

INDEX